Agents of
Bacterial Disease

Agents of Bacterial Disease

ALBERT S. KLAINER, M.D.

Professor of Medicine
Chairman, Division of Infectious Diseases
West Virginia University School of Medicine
Morgantown, West Virginia

IRVING GEIS

New York City, N.Y.

Medical Department
Harper & Row, Publishers
Hagerstown, Maryland
New York, Evanston, San Francisco, London

DEDICATION

To my wife, Jo-Ann,
whose love and encouragement
played an immeasurable role
in the writing of this book.

A.S.K.

Contents

Foreword

A true *understanding* of the clinical features of disease is based on an awareness and application of all available specific information concerning the pathogenesis, pathophysiology, and pathoanatomy of a particular disorder. It is interesting in this regard that in only a few of the very large number of diseases that affect man are the responsible mechanisms so well defined that they permit a highly accurate prediction of the nature and course of uncomplicated and complicated disease. So, while the clinical syndromes and pathologic changes associated with atherosclerosis are well known, its etiology and pathophysiologic mechanisms are still subjects of controversy. This is true even for some of the common infections. Thus, while the etiology of staphylococcal infection is firmly established, it is presently not at all clear what actually transpires in the affected patient. Despite the availability of increasing information concerning the type and nature of a number of toxins elaborated by *Staphylococcus aureus*, the manner in which these act to alter function in man and contribute to the clinical disturbances produced by this organism is not well understood. The situation is similar with respect to tuberculosis. Here again the etiology of the disease is completely defined, and many of the individual components of the tubercle bacillus have been isolated and identified. Despite this knowledge and definition of the characteristic pathologic changes, the pathophysiologic mechanisms involved in tuberculosis are still not totally understood.

The application of information concerning the exact mechanisms involved to an analysis of the clinical features of an infection makes it possible not only to understand the basis of many, if not all, of its manifestations, but also to predict its natural history. Several infections illustrate this clearly. It is a well-known fact that the basic lesion of subacute bacterial endocarditis is a sterile platelet–fibrin thrombus present on the endocardium of a valve previously altered by a disease such as rheumatic fever. Formation of the thrombus is induced by "whipping out" of platelets and fibrin as blood passes over the roughened surface of the abnormal valve leaflet, the site on which organisms are implanted during the course of a transient bacteremia. Agglutinating antibody specific for the organism must be present in order for a large enough inoculum to settle out on the thrombus to allow initiation of growth and infection. In subacute endocarditis, the pathologic features are those consistent with a process in which both healing and destruction proceed simultaneously at a slow rate, the healing not quite catching up with the destruction. This accounts for the prolonged course of the disease. In those instances in which blood cultures are negative, it is now clear that this is due to the presence of specific bactericidal antibody. Even one of the common complications of this disease, glomerulonephritis, is now completely understood since it has been demonstrated to be due to the deposition of immune complexes in the basement membrane of the glomerulus. The manifestations of scarlet fever in the skin (typical rash) and kidney are readily explained on the basis of the known pathophysiologic effects of the erythrogenic toxin elaborated by the streptococci that cause this disease. This toxin is a capillary poison that induces dilatation, congestion, and increased fragility of the capillary bed. Diffuse dilatation of these vessels results in generalized erythema of the skin; congestion of the capillary tuft in the papillae of the skin produces the red punctate component of the rash; increased fragility of the capillaries leads to the development of the bleeding lines (Pastia's lines), a positive tourniquet test, and an increase in the number of red blood cells in the urine. In the same manner, most of the clinical manifestations of tetanus are now easily understood because the pathophysiology of the disease has been well worked out. Tetanospasmin, the toxin responsible for this disorder, acts on four areas of the nervous system, dysfunction of which is responsible for all of the features of the syndrome. The localized muscle phenomena are due to interference by the toxin with neuromuscular transmission by inhibiting the release of acetylcholine from nerve terminals in the muscle. The characteristic convulsive seizures that characterize this disease are due to action on the spinal cord that leads to dysfunction of polysynaptic reflexes involving interneurones and resulting in inhibition of antagonists. The antidromic inhibition of evoked cerebral cortical activity is reduced. Involvement of the sympathetic nervous system results in the development of labile hypertension, tachycardia, peripheral vasoconstriction, cardiac arrhythmias, profuse sweating, and increased urinary excretion of catecholamines. These examples illustrate clearly the ease with which the clinical pictures of some infectious processes are readily explained and understood once the basic mechanisms involved in their production have been defined.

This book furnishes the basic information concerning bacterial morphology, biochemistry, and physiology that should allow the reader to understand the phenomena involved in the pathogenesis and clinical behavior of some infectious diseases as well as the effects that antimicrobial agents have on their etiologic agents. It is only by this approach that students of disease can gain a valid understanding of the reasons for the development of some, if not all, of the manifestations of a given disorder and, on this basis, plan the most effective attacks not only in the area of diagnosis but also of treatment.

Louis Weinstein, Ph.D., M.D.

Preface

This introductory text presents a unique visual approach to the study of the common bacteria which cause human disease. In the standard textbook, illustrations are usually employed to complement, strengthen, reinforce, exemplify or embellish vital textual material; thus the assimilation of information is almost wholly dependent on retention of the written word. In this book, the converse is true. Learning is primarily visual—the illustrations form the heart of the matter, with the text describing, explaining, and expanding upon what is shown. Hopefully this approach will provide the beginning student of bacteriology with a more comfortable introduction to the subject than has heretofore been available.

Numerous scanning electronphotomicrographs provide a unique means of demonstrating microorganisms and bacteriologic phenomena in three dimensions at high magnification. Together with detailed diagrammatic illustrations, these photomicrographs allow rapid assimilation of the material with a minimum of effort and textual material.

In addition, a number of full page diagrams form an integral part of the communication process by serving as concise visual summaries of the corresponding text. These schematic visual presentations are virtually autonomous in that their coverage of broad topics in bacteriology is not dependent on the text.

Throughout the book, emphasis is placed on the pathogenesis and mechanisms of bacterial diseases and on the relation of bacteriology to clinical infectious diseases. No attempt has been made to write a comprehensive textbook covering all of the bacteria which cause diseases in humans; rather, subjects lending themselves to illustration and serving to introduce the broad groups of bacteria to the beginning student are emphasized, offering the student a solid background in bacteriology and an introduction to the clinical significance of bacteria–human disease—in a format that can be easily read and understood.

The authors wish to express their appreciation to the staff of Harper and Row Publishers for their untiring efforts in the production of this book, as well as their unfailing patience and constant encouragement in the preparation of the final manuscript.

The authors are especially grateful to Dr. Louis Weinstein, Professor of Medicine, Chief, Infectious Disease Service, Tufts–New England Medical Center Hospitals, Boston, Massachusetts, not only for writing the Foreword, but because it was his lifelong devotion to excellence in teaching and his constant awareness of students' problems in learning that stimulated us to prepare this text.

A.S.K.
I.G.

Agents of
Bacterial Disease

1

Structure and Morphology of Bacteria

Bacteria are a heterogeneous group of microscopic unicellular organisms. Although the thousands of species are differentiated by many factors, including morphology, staining reactions, nutritional requirements, metabolism, and antigenic structure, individual cells and groups of cells have certain morphologic characteristics and spatial relations in common.

STRUCTURE OF BACTERIAL CELLS
Surface Structure

Bacteria may be surrounded by as many as three surface layers: 1) capsule or slime layer, 2) cell wall, and 3) cell membrane (Figs. 1-1 through 1-3).

Capsule or Slime Layer

The outermost layer is a low-density, viscous envelope; it is called a capsule when it is well defined and a slime layer when it is less so. Not all bacteria possess this layer; some have capsules only under certain cultural conditions and during certain stages of growth. The size and characteristics of the capsule vary widely from strain to strain, but the capsule is usually a gelatinous polymer of polysaccharide, polypeptide, or both, of varying complexity. In some species, such as *Pneumococcus* and *Klebsiella pneumoniae*,

1

Fig. 1–1.
A. Major surface layers of a bacterium, in this case a rod-shaped microorganism or a bacillus.
B. Section of a bacillus demonstrating the major anatomic features.

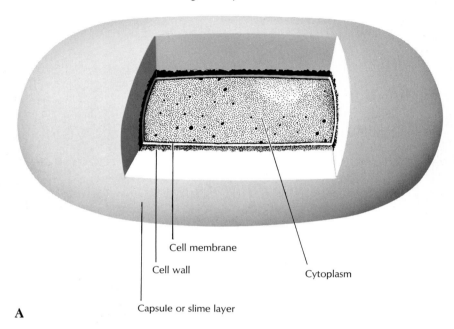

Cell membrane

Cell wall

Cytoplasm

Capsule or slime layer

A

B

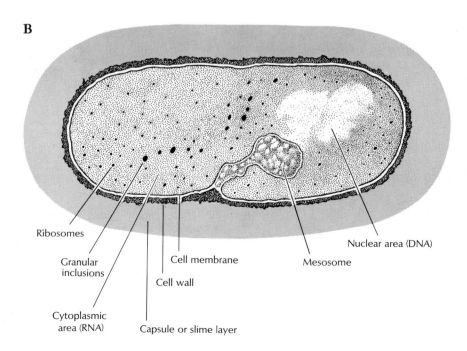

Ribosomes

Granular
inclusions

Cell membrane

Cell wall

Nuclear area (DNA)

Mesosome

Cytoplasmic
area (RNA)

Capsule or slime layer

Fig. 1–2.
Transmission electron micrograph of a group of *Staphylococcus aureus*, demonstrating the cell wall (A), cell membrane (B), mesosome (C), transverse septum (D), nucleoid (E), ribosomes (F), and storage granules (G). (×60,000)

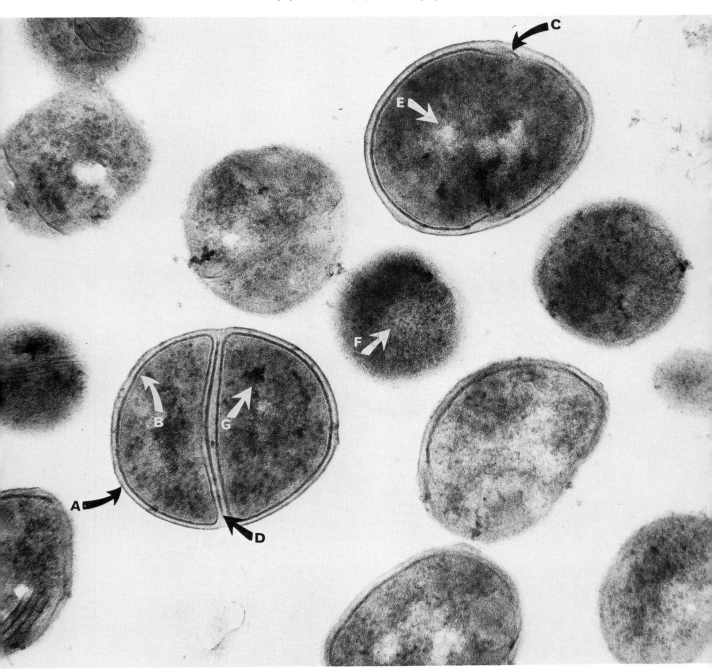

Fig. 1–3.
Scanning electron micrograph of *Escherichia coli,*
demonstrating the cell wall (A), cell membrane
(B), site of transverse septum formation (C), and
cytoplasm (D). (×10,000)

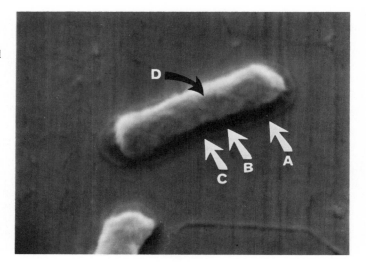

it may be thicker than the diameter of the cell; in others it is barely visible even with special stains. The exact structural relation of the capsule to the remainder of the cell is not known. The capsule is thought to be of intracellular origin, excreted by the cell and adhering to the surface because of its viscous properties.

The capsule can be visualized by several methods: 1) capsular stains; 2) simple India ink suspensions in which the capsule appears as a clear zone between the opaque medium and the cell itself; and 3) in the case of some species, specific anticapsular antibodies which enhance visualization by causing the capsule to swell (the Quellung reaction, described in Chapter 5, *Pneumococci,* is typical of this phenomenon).

Although the capsular layer is not indispensible to the bacterial cell, it is of potential value. In pathogenic bacteria, virulence may be related to the presence of a capsule which protects the cell from phagocytosis; the loss of the capsule may result in a parallel loss of virulence.

Cell Wall   The cell wall (Figs. 1-1 through 1-3) is a complex, semirigid structure which helps to maintain the overall integrity of the cell as well as its characteristic size and shape. It surrounds the cell membrane, protecting it and the cytoplasm within from adverse changes in the environment, especially alterations in osmotic forces. Although the cell wall maintains the general shape of bacteria exposed to hypo- or hypertonic environments, the surface topography may change (Fig. 1-4). If the wall of a bacterium is damaged or removed, significant morphologic alterations occur. Weakening or destroying the bacterial cell wall with lysozyme, or inhibiting cell wall synthesis with penicillin, may kill bacteria by rendering them incapable of preserving the normal equilibrium between the intra- and extracellular environments; if the external environment is hypotonic the cell bursts, but if the plasma membrane is stabilized by keeping the organism in hypertonic solution the cell may survive in this altered state (Fig. 1-5). It is of interest

Fig. 1–4.

Alterations in the surface topography of bacteria due to changes in the tonicity of the environment; the organism is *Proteus vulgaris*.

A. Exposed to water, the organism appears full and the surface smooth.

B. Exposed to 0.9% NaCl, the organism develops the appearance of a leaf-like ellipsoid due to shrinkage.

C. Exposed to 15% sucrose, the organism exhibits plasmolysis or shrinkage of the cytoplasm from the cell membrane causing flattening of the ends. The fine, thread-like structures in the background are flagella. (×10,000)

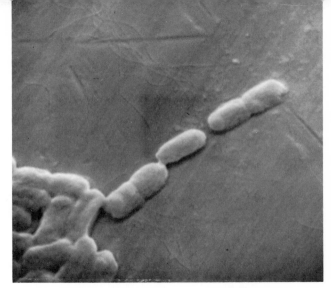

A

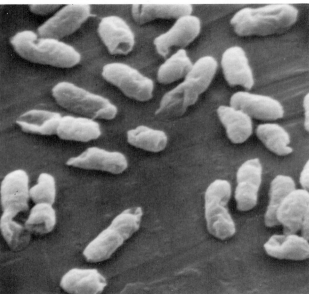

B
C

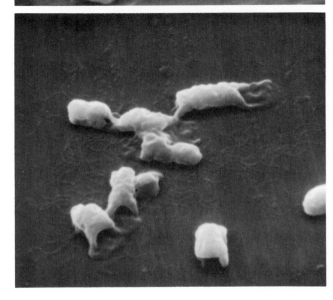

Fig. 1–5.

Effect of lysozyme on a bacillus. Lysozyme causes cell wall defects which allow extrusion of intracellular material. In the absence of cell wall integrity, the cell is incapable of preserving equilibrium between the intra- and extracellular environments; it then swells, with the resulting structure being a spheroplast (or cell wall-defective organism). If the external environment is hypotonic, the cell swells and ruptures, leaving behind cellular debris and membrane-like structures thought to be collapsed spheroplasts. If the external environment is hypertonic, the cell membrane is stabilized, and the cell may survive as a spheroplast.

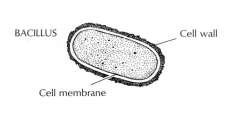

BACILLUS   Cell wall

Cell membrane

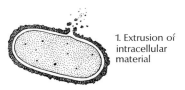

1. Extrusion of intracellular material

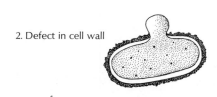

2. Defect in cell wall

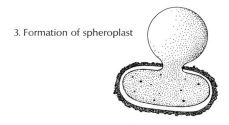

3. Formation of spheroplast

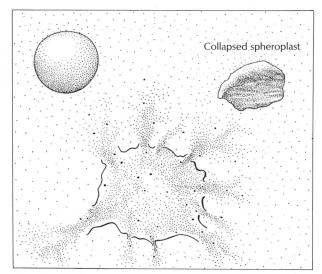

Collapsed spheroplast

Hypotonic environment

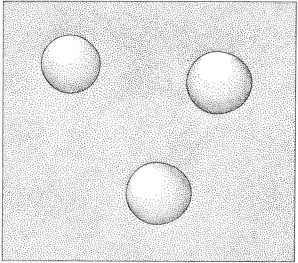

Hypertonic environment

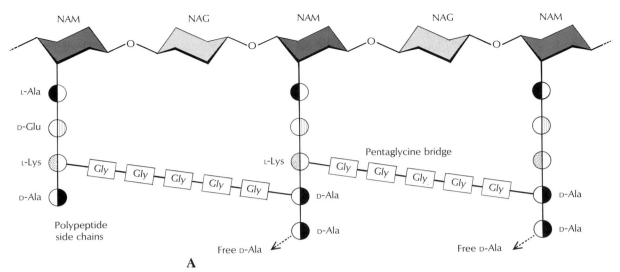

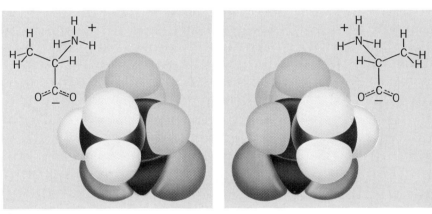

Fig. 1–6.
Structural composition of the innermost basal layer of the bacterial cell wall.
A. The main chain of the mucopeptide layer is an alternating copolymer of N-acetylglucosamine (NAG) and N-acetylmuramic acid (NAM) units. The side chains of NAM units are linked by pentaglycine bridges. This example is taken from the cell wall of *Staphylococcus aureus*.
B. Both L-alanine and its mirror image D-alanine are found in the mucopeptide layer of cell walls.
(Illustration **B** from Dickerson RE, Geis I: The Structure and Action of Proteins. Menlo Park, Calif, WA Benjamin, 1969, © Dickerson and Geis.)

that although bacteria have a variety of shapes, they are usually round if their cell walls are damaged or removed, because the weak, flexible plasma membrane assumes the spherical shape for maximum stability.

Although the cell walls of gram-positive and gram-negative bacteria are not identical, the structural compositions of their innermost basal layers are similar (Fig. 1-6). The basal layer or backbone of the cell wall is composed of a three-dimensional network of mucopeptides, the basic components of which are two simple sugars and three or four amino acids.

The two sugars (glucosamine and muramic acid) are related to glucose. Glucosamine, an amino sugar, is a common constituent of natural polymers, e.g., chitin and cellulose, and is in the form of N-acetylglucosamine in the bacterial cell wall. Muramic acid is a lactic acid derivative of glucosamine found only in bacteria and microorganisms that resemble bacteria, such as the blue-green algae; like glucosamine it is usually in the form of the N-acetyl derivative. These sugars are present in polysaccharide chains of various lengths consisting of alternating N-acetylglucosamine and N-acetyl-muramic acid units joined together by $1 \rightarrow 4$ β—glycoside linkages.

Only a limited number of amino acids are found in the cell wall: glutamic acid, glycine, lysine, and alanine. Glutamic acid is found in the usually D stereoisomeric configuration; lysine has the usual L configuration; alanine is found as both the D and L stereoisomers. Many bacteria have no lysine in the cell wall; instead the wall contains diaminopimelic acid, whose structure resembles that of lysine; diaminopimelic acid is peculiar to the bacterial cell wall and is not found in any protein. The amino acids of the cell wall are linked by peptide bonds to form polypeptides.

In general, then, the basic structure of the inner mucopeptide layer of the cell wall of both gram-positive and gram-negative bacteria consists of polysaccharide chains of alternating N-acetylglucosamine and N-acetyl-muramic acid units. Attached to and cross linking the polysaccharide chains are peptides linked to one another by pentaglycine bridges. The polypeptide cross links differ from one species of microorganism to another but generally do not contain more than four different amino acids. D-Alanine and D-glutamic acid seem always to be present.

The wall of a gram-positive bacterium is a thick (150–800 nm), uniformly dense layer in close apposition to the cell membrane. The inner or basal layer is the three-dimensional mucopeptide described above. It is associated with other components, especially teichoic acids (polymers of ribitol phosphate or of glycerol phosphate) and/or mucopolysaccharides.

In gram-negative bacteria the basal mucopeptide layer is covered by outer layers of lipopolysaccharide and lipoprotein. The linkage between the inner mucopeptide layer and the outer lipopolysaccharide layer is unclear. The cell walls of gram-negative bacteria do not contain teichoic acids. The lipopolysaccharide layer is of particular importance because it is primarily responsible for the somatic O antigenic specificity of gram-negative bacteria and because it is intimately related to endotoxicity.

Cell Membrane   The cell membrane (cytoplasmic membrane) is a thin functional structure that surrounds the cytoplasm of the cell and separates it from the inner surface of the cell wall (Figs. 1-1 through 1-3). It is a triple-layered unit membrane too thin to be seen by light microscopy. Transmission electron microscopy has shown it as two dark bands separated by a light band. It is a complex lipoprotein (about 40% lipid and 60% protein with small amounts of carbohydrate) similar to the cell membrane of mammalian cells, except that it contains little or no phosphatidyl choline and no sterols (except in certain mycoplasmal organisms).

The cell membrane is the site of several enzyme systems, including the cytochrome system, as well as those of succinic dehydrogenase, lactic dehydrogenase, and acid phosphatase; the membrane serves many of the functions that mitochondria perform in higher plants and animals. Most important, however, it is a semipermeable, selective membrane that governs the passage of materials into and out of the cell via the many different transport systems it contains and by acting as an osmotic barrier.

Fig. 1–7.
Transport mechanisms across the cell membrane.

MOVEMENT OF SUBSTANCES ACROSS CELL MEMBRANES

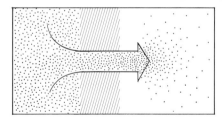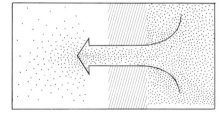

Osmosis
From higher
to lower
concentration

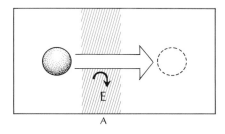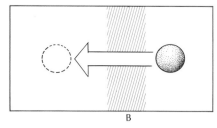

A

B

Active transport (A)
requires energy (E).
Passive transport (B)
does not require
energy.

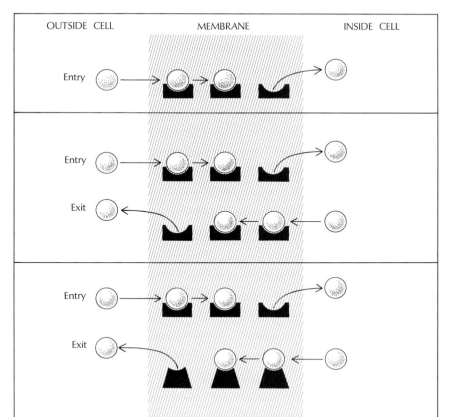

OUTSIDE CELL   MEMBRANE   INSIDE CELL

Entry

Carrier protein
for transporting
molecules across
cell membranes

Entry

Exit

Homologous
system uses same
carrier protein for
entry and exit

Entry

Exit

Heterologous
system uses *different*
carrier protein for
entry and exit

Movement of substances across the cell membrane in either direction generally occurs by means of active transport, passive transport, and osmosis and diffusion from a higher to a lower concentration (Fig. 1-7). If the external environment of a cell becomes hypotonic, water flows into the cell causing it to swell; if the environment is made hypertonic, water flows out of the cell causing it to shrink. This phenomenon is a relatively simple process dependent on the concentration of water inside and outside the cell and on the permeability of the cell membrane to water. For many substances this simple osmotic relation does not exist, thus protecting the cell from the indiscriminate flow of substances across its membrane. On the other hand, the uptake of various substances can be induced or repressed by altering the growth medium of bacteria; this phenomenon is related to the formation of specific transport systems rather than to changes in the permeability of the cell membrane. In fact, such transport systems resemble enzymes and are frequently called permeases. The cell membrane also contains preexisting transport systems which are classified as "active" (requiring the expenditure of energy) or "passive" (not requiring the expenditure of energy). Most transport systems display specificity for specific individual or structurally related compounds. Specific transport systems have been demonstrated for several sugars and amino acids, although the structural and functional characteristics of systems for these two classes of compounds differ. Theoretically some transport systems function via carrier or transport proteins which "carry" substances across the cell membrane (Fig. 1-7).

In contrast to entry into cells, most substances are thought to exit from cells by nonspecific diffusion through pores in the cell membrane; this is accomplished in a fashion dependent on the internal concentration of the substance in much the same way as water enters and leaves the cell. Nevertheless, evidence is accumulating that specific transport systems may exist or those used for entry may be used for exit as well. Most transport systems for exit are probably homologous to those for entry; heterologous systems, however, may be present.

Careful electron microscopic examination of ultrathin sections of bacteria shows occasional irregular invaginations of the cytoplasmic membrane. These are called mesosomes (Fig. 1-2). Depending upon the plane of the section examined, they may appear as vesicles or as isolated, concentric lamellar bodies; they are always connected to and part of the cell membrane. Mesosomes increase the surface area of the cell membrane and thereby aid in diffusion or transport. Their frequent proximity to the nuclear region of the cell and the transverse septum (Figs. 1-2 and 1-3) observed during cell division suggests that they may play a role in cell wall synthesis and the partition of cellular material during the formation of daughter cells. Thus although the cell membrane contributes little to the size and shape of the cell, its structural and functional integrity are of the utmost importance for the cell to exist in its normal state.

Cytoplasmic Structure   That part of the cell surrounded by the cell membrane is called the cytoplasm (Figs. 1-1 and 1-3). It is much less complex than the cytoplasm of mammalian cells and can be arbitrarily divided into three compartments: 1) the cytoplasmic area, which is rich in ribonucleic acid (RNA); 2) the nuclear area, which is rich in deoxyribonucleic acid (DNA); and 3) the fluid component, which is about 80% water and contains a myriad of small molecules and inorganic ions.

The cytoplasmic area appears finely granular because of the presence of ribosomes (Fig. 1-2); these are spherical structures 150–200 nm in diameter which contain about 90% of the RNA of the bacterial cell and are not membrane-bound in bacteria. Ribosomes play a major role in protein synthesis and during this process form chains called polyribosomes. Because ribosomes are densely packed throughout the cytoplasmic area, they cannot be identified readily as specific structures in sectioned bacteria. The cytoplasmic area also contains a number of granular inclusions which basically are storage granules (Fig. 1-2). Such reserves of polymetaphosphates stain metachromatically and are called volutin granules; others contain lipids (such as polyhydroxybutyric acid), glycogen, granulose (a starch-like polymer of glucose), or sulfur. The polysaccharide and lipid granules are generally considered to represent endproducts of metabolism and play no active role in the physiology of the cell. The volutin granules represent sites of enzyme activity; the polymetaphosphates are a source of high-energy phosphate bonds accumulated during oxidative phosphorylation via adenosine triphosphate (ATP).

The nucleus of a bacterium is not surrounded by a nuclear membrane and lacks discrete chromosomes, mitotic apparatus, and a nucleolus. Hence it is simply a nuclear region (Fig. 1-2) which is sometimes called the chromatin body, nucleoid or nuclear equivalent. It can be seen by light microscopy with special strains or by phase-contrast microscopy under appropriate refractive conditions. The nuclear region generally occupies a central position in the cell; its shape varies from a sphere to an elongated, irregular, dumbbell-like structure. Under electron microscopy it appears to consist of parallel, curved bundles of delicate fibers thought to be strands of DNA. Despite these structural differences from the nucleus of eucaryotic cells, its functions are similar.

Flagella   Flagella are the organs of locomotion for the microorganisms that possess them (Fig. 1-8). They are thin, filamentous appendages composed almost entirely of elastic protein (flagellin) and attached to both the cell wall and the cytoplasmic membrane by a granule, the basal body. In *Escherichia coli* the basal body consists of two pairs of rings mounted on a rod; it is proximal to that part of the flagellum called the hook. (Although most of the flagellum is uniform in shape, it has a hook-like appearance and a slight constriction near the attachment to the basal body.) The structural attachment of the flagellum can be visualized as follows (Fig. 1-9): The L-ring of the basal body specifically is attached to the lipopolysaccharide layer, the P-ring to the mucopeptide layer, and the M-ring to the cytoplasmic membrane; above the M-ring is an S-ring which does not appear to be attached to any specific structure. Each ring seems to be a chemically distinct component of the basal body, but the chemistry remains to be elucidated. This model of flagellar attachment is applicable to most gram-negative bacteria; in gram-positive bacteria the basal body clearly functions to anchor a

Fig. 1–8.
Proteus vulgaris as seen by scanning electron microscopy. Flagella are seen as fine, thread-like structures in the background. (×30,000)

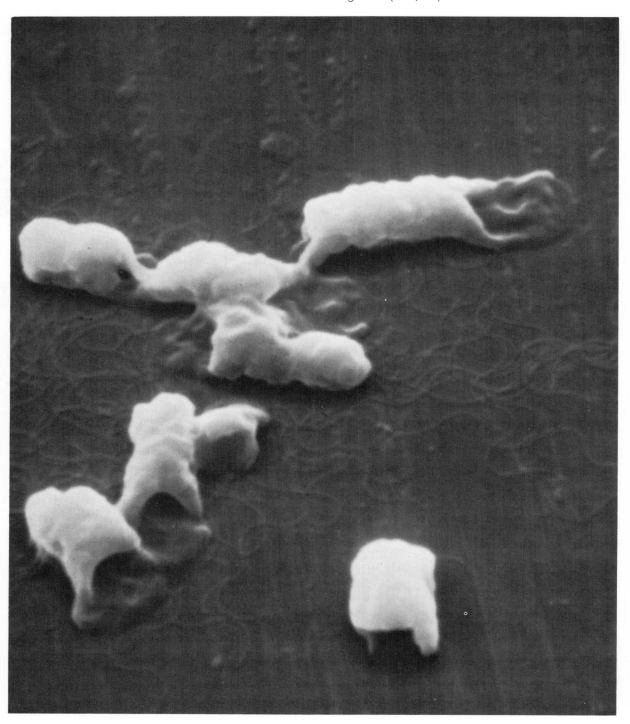

Fig. 1–9.
Structural attachment of flagella.

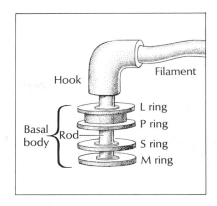

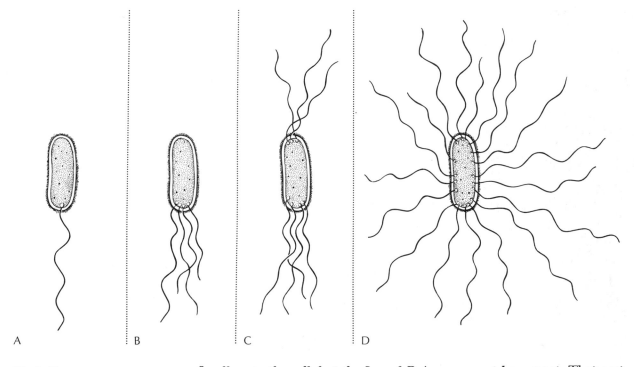

flagellum to the cell, but the L- and P-rings may not be present. That part of the flagellum external to the cell is a thin (100–200 nm), wavy, hair-like structure which does not taper and is of variable length (1–70 μ, average 15–25 μ).

Flagella can be visualized by darkfield microscopy; to be seen by ordinary light microscopy, they must be coated with special flagellar stains. Although the number of flagella varies widely, the pattern of flagellation is a genetically stable characteristic. Four types of arrangement are common (Fig. 1-10): monotrichous (single polar flagellum), lopotrichous (two or more flagella at one pole of the cell), amphitrichous (tufts of flagella at both ends of the cell), and peritrichous (flagella distributed over the entire cell). Flagella are seen in many species of bacilli but rarely in cocci.

Flagella are coiled in the form of cylindrical helices. The ultrastructure consists of subunits of flagellin which aggregate to form a hollow cylindrical structure. They are too thin, however, to contain the nine peripheral and two central subfibrils found in the cilia of higher forms.

The number of flagella determines the vigor of the movement of bacteria. Extremely large numbers of flagella endow bacteria (e.g., *Proteus*) with an ability to "swarm" in a thin film over the surface of some solid culture media. The movement of bacteria probably results from metabolic activity in the basal body imparted to the filamentous portion of the flagella and resulting in a wavelike action. It should be remembered, however, that certain bacteria move by other means, e.g., spirochetes by contraction of their helical structure around a more rigid axial filament, and some slime bacteria by a gliding mechanism.

Flagella are antigenically distinct from the rest of the cell and elicit specific antiflagellar antibodies. In the presence of specific antibody, flagella are agglutinated and their function is impaired; bacteria are thus immobilized.

Pili (Fimbriae)

Pili or fimbriae are minute, filamentous appendages composed of protein subunits and visualized only by electron microscopy. Fimbriae are smaller, shorter, less rigid, and more numerous than flagella and do not form regular waves; like flagella, however, they appear to arise from basal bodies in the cytoplasmic membrane. They may be present in nonmotile as well as motile bacteria and are thought to function as organs of attachment rather than motility. In some bacteria, "sex" pili play an essential role in the attachment of conjugating cells; the "male" cell has one or two hollow pili that apparently form a bridge with the "female" cell for the transfer of DNA.

Spores

Gram-positive bacilli, the aerobes of the genus *Bacillus*, and the anaerobic clostridia exhibit the ability to form endospores under certain environmental conditions. Spores are spherical or ovoid structures composed of a spore coat, a cortex, and a nuclear core. They are produced intracellularly (hence the name endospores) and are smaller than the parent cell, although the diameter of the spore may be larger or smaller than that of the vegetative (metabolically active) parent cell. Generally a single cell produces one spore, which may be located centrally, terminally, or subterminally depending on the species (Fig. 1-11). Although metabolically less active than the precursor cell, spores do manifest metabolic activity; they also contain enzymes of the nonglycolytic shunt and the tricarboxylic acid cycle as well as an electron-transport system. All bacterial spores contain large amounts of dipicolinic acid (a substance not found in vegetative cells) and calcium, which together form a complex located in the outer spore membrane.

The factors leading to spore formation are poorly understood; in general, spores are formed under conditions unfavorable for growth. When spore formation occurs, it is generally at the end of or just following the phase of exponential growth. At the start of spore formation, light microscopy reveals a localized area of increased density—the forespore—which may develop the appearance of an enlarging granule and from which the highly refractile spore is formed. When the spore has developed, the surrounding vegetative cell sloughs off. Visualized by the transmission electron microscope, a spore is formed by invagination of the cell membrane around a chromosome and a small amount of cytoplasm; this sequestered portion of the cell ultimately develops into the spore.

Under certain conditions, usually those more favorable for growth, the spore germinates to form one vegetative cell. Germination consists of three stages: 1) activation (although some bacterial spores germinate spontaneously, others must be activated by certain stimuli such as heat or aging); 2) germination (the uptake of water); and 3) outgrowth (the spore core grows, the vegetative wall develops, and the vegetative cell bursts out of the spore coat). During germination, the refractile appearance of the spore changes, and it again develops the characteristics of a vegetative cell. The spore may become thin and stretch into the shape of the vegetative cell, or a vegetative cell may appear to grow within the spore wall, which ultimately splits and is discarded. The morphology of germination varies, the vegetative cell protruding through one side of the spore wall or at one or both ends. In any case, since only one vegetative cell is produced, germination is not a means of multiplication.

The true biologic function of the spore is not known, but spores exhibit significant resistance to heating, freezing, drying, irradiation, and exposure to noxious chemicals. Resistance to heat is thought to be related to the calcium dipicolinate complex, which may stabilize cellular proteins against unfolding by denaturation. The mechanism of resistance to stains and disinfectants such as phenol, however, is probably related to the spore's impermeability to these substances. Teleologically speaking, then, spores represent a state of latency or suspended metabolic activity which may protect bacteria from harm.

GROSS MORPHOLOGY   Although knowledge of the structure of the bacterial cell is basic to the study of bacteriology, and the transmission of electron microscope has provided a means of correlating ultrastructure with cell biochemistry and physiology, the gross morphology of individual cells and their spatial relations to one another as viewed with the light microscope are still of practical significance. The ultimate identity of a bacterium is determined by many parameters, most of which are dependent on culture. In many instances, however, the tentative identity of a microorganism must be determined without the delay inherent in cultural methods; this is especially true, for example, when the presence of a life-threatening infectious disease dictates that appropriate therapy be chosen and administered before the results of culture are available. In these instances, examination of smears of clinical material may provide immediate information about the microorganisms involved. Also serial examination of smears from cultures helps give meaningful direction to the laboratory identification of microorganisms. It should be emphasized, however, that even in the hands of the most experienced microbiologist, identification of gross morphology is a method of tentative diagnosis and no more.

Individual bacteria have one of three general shapes: spherical, rod-shaped, or spiral.

Fig. 1–11.
Spores of a species of *Clostridium* as seen by scanning electron microscopy.
A. Vegetative cell.
B. Central spore.
(*Continued*)

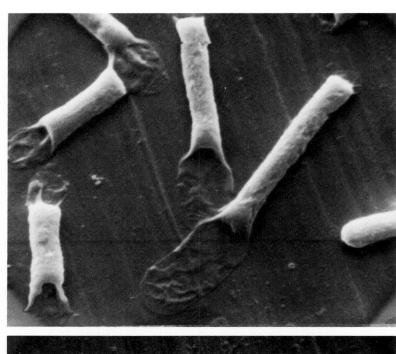

A

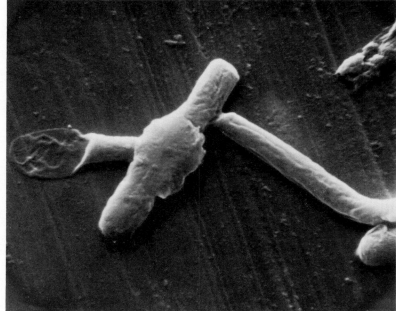

B

Spherical bacteria are termed cocci and may be truly spherical (e.g., staphylococci), lancet- or helmet-shaped (e.g., pneumococci), or kidney- or bean-shaped (e.g., neisseriae), as seen in Figure 1-12. Cocci are usually visualized in certain characteristic spatial relations to one another (Fig. 1-13).

(*Fig. 1–11, continued*)
C. Terminal spore.
D. Subterminal spore.
(×10,000)

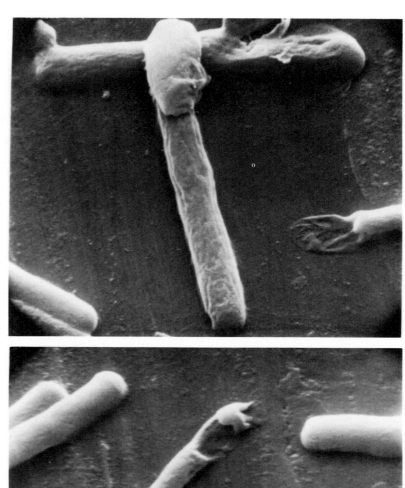

C

D

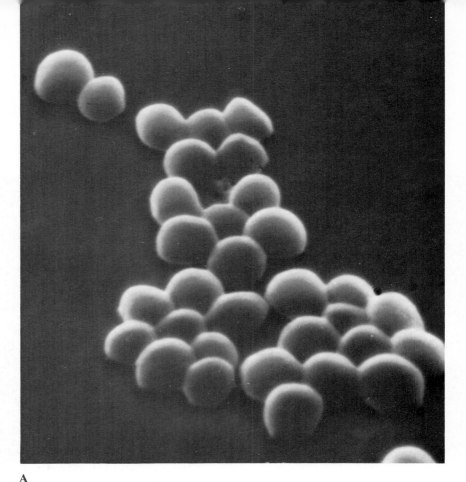

Fig. 1–12.
Spherical bacteria.
A. Staphylococci.
B. Pneumococci.
C. Neisseriae.
(×10,000)

A

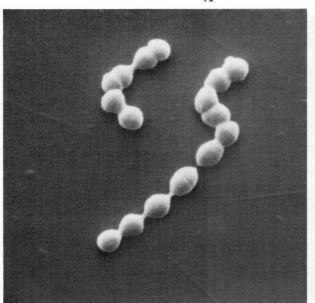
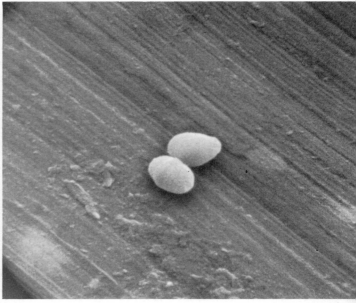

B C

Fig. 1–13.
Spatial relationships of cocci.
A. Cocci seen singly, paired, and in a chain.
B. Triad.
C. Tetrad.
D. Clusters.
(×10,000)

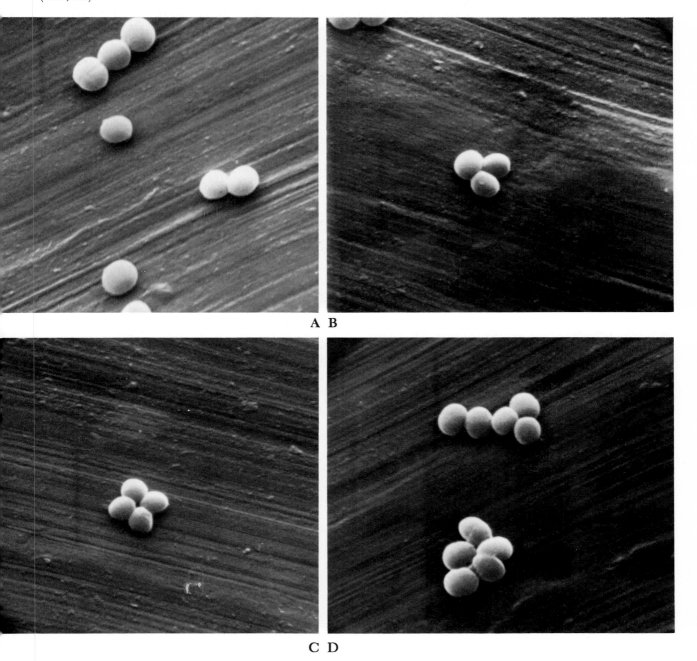

A B

C D

Fig. 1–14.
Axes of the spherical shaped
bacteria, demonstrating the
parallel short axes of
pneumococci, parallel long
axes of neisseriae, and equal
axes of staphylococci and
streptococci.

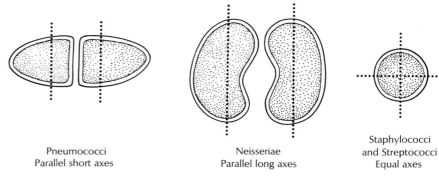

Pneumococci
Parallel short axes

Neisseriae
Parallel long axes

Staphylococci
and Streptococci
Equal axes

Spatial arrangement of cocci:

1. Singly.

2. In pairs: diplococci. Characteristically, pneumococci and neisseriae are diplococci. Although the former are lancet-shaped and gram-positive, and the latter kidney-shaped and gram-negative, they are occasionally variable in shape and staining characteristics. In this situation they may be identified by the fact that the short axes of pneumococci are parallel; in contrast, the long axes of neisseriae are parallel, and the axes of truly spherical cocci are equal (Fig. 1-14).

3. In rows or chains: streptococci. Diplococci, especially pneumococci, however, may arrange themselves end-to-end and appear to form chains.

4. In threes: triads.

5. In fours: tetrads.

6. In cuboidal pockets of eight cells: sarcinae.

7. In grape-like clusters: staphylococci.

These spatial arrangements can be explained by the planes in which cocci multiply (Fig. 1-15). Bacteria multiply predominantly by binary fission, one cell dividing transversely to produce two new cells. If a single coccus divides in one plane, diplococci or streptococci result. Cocci that divide in two planes at right angles to one another result in tetrads. If cocci divide in three planes at right angles to one another, cubes or packets of cells are formed. Although the spatial arrangement of cocci may be typical of particular species of bacteria, not all cells of a species are necessarily arranged in this way. For example, staphylococci may appear as single cells, diplococci, triads, or short chains, or any grouping of cells may separate from the typical grape-like cluster.

Rod-shaped bacteria are designated bacilli (Fig. 1-16). Although the typical arrangement of cocci is not characteristic of the bacilli, occasionally the latter do appear in pairs (diplobacilli) or end-to-end in what appear to be chains (streptobacilli). In addition, certain species form characteristic spatial patterns, e.g., the picket-fence or palisade arrangement or cuneiform figures of *Corynebacterium diphtheriae*. Like cocci, however, bacilli vary in morphology, especially in the relation of their width and length, so that bacilli of varying length, coccobacilli, and filamentous forms are typical of some species.

One plane (pairs)

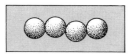  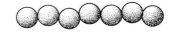

One plane (chains)

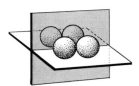 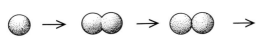 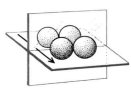

Two planes (four cells)

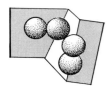 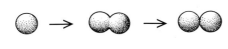   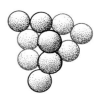

Three planes (irregular pattern, bunches)

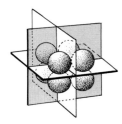 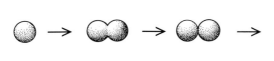 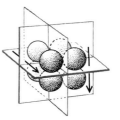

Three planes (regular pattern, cuboidal arrangement)

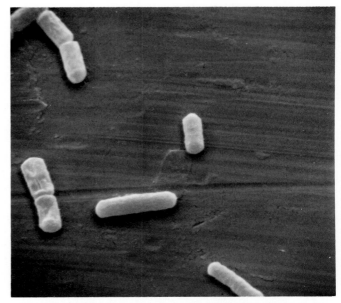

Fig. 1–17.
Treponema pallidum, a typical spirochete.
(×10,000)

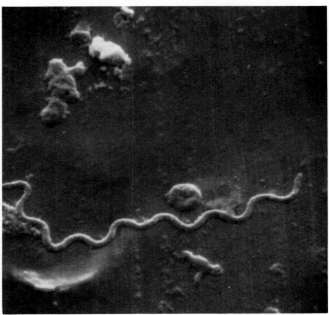

The spirochetes of syphilis exemplify the spiral-shaped bacteria (Fig. 1-17). Other spirilla are characterized by their length, number, and amplitude of spirals, as well as the nature of their coils. Short, incomplete spirals are comma-shaped, e.g., vibrios.

Although these are the most typical shapes and spatial configurations of bacteria, there are other bacterial forms whose specific morphology must be learned as each is studied.

Table 1-1. Differential Features of Smooth and Rough Colonies

Feature	Smooth colony	Rough colony
Colonial morphology	Smooth, convex, viscous	Irregular, flat, dry
Virulence	Pathogenic forms virulent	Pathogenic forms avirulent
Presence of capsules in encapsulated species	Capsules present	Capsules absent or diminished
Antigenicity	Complete	Often lost; occasionally new antigens present

Although individual bacterial cells can be seen only with the aid of a microscope, the bacterial colony—presumably the product of multiplication of a single organism on solid media—is a macroscopic structural entity with specific morphologic characteristics. Colonies are described in terms of diameter and size, nature of their margins (regular or irregular), shape (circular or ovoid), elevation (flat, raised, thin, or thick), color (pigmented or nonpigmented), and whether they are opaque, translucent, or opalescent.

One of the most important features of a colony is its surface texture. Rough (R) colonies have a dry, flat, irregular, wrinkled appearance and are generally formed by cells that lack a capsule. Smooth (S) colonies are convex, round, and shiny and are usually regarded as the "normal" form. Intermediate (SR and RS) forms are also seen; transformation of an S colony into an R colony probably is via the SR and RS intermediate forms. The M (mucoid) colony is a third commonly recognized type and may be associated with both S and R colonies. The relation between the types of colonies can be summarized as follows: S has a constant tendency to change to R; the reverse is more difficult. The differential features of S and R colonies are presented in Table 1-1. There are exceptions to these general differences. The basis for S to R transformation is not the same for all species, but it is dependent mainly on genetic and environmental factors. Most important, however, is that this remarkable example of bacterial variation—in fact the overall morphology of bacterial colonies—is mainly a function of the morphology of the individual cells that make up the colony.

SUGGESTED READING

1. DAVIS BD, DULBECCO R, EISEN HN, et al: Microbiology. Second edition. Hagerstown, Md., Harper and Row, 1973, pp 21–58

2. WEIBULL C: Morphology and chemical anatomy of bacteria, Bacterial and Mycotic Infections in Man. Fourth edition. Edited by R J Dubos and J G Hirsch. Philadelphia, Lippincott, 1965, pp 37–71

2

Pertinent Aspects of Bacteriology

Examination of bacteria involves a variety of related and unrelated techniques, the ultimate goal of which is identification. Individual bacteria, or suspensions or smears of bacteria, are examined visually with the aid of the microscope, the instrumentation and complexity of which determine the limits of magnification and the information that can be obtained (Table 2-1). Further isolation and ultimate identification is dependent on cultural techniques based upon the nutritional requirements and biochemical reactions of microorganisms and the use of media which selectively enhance or inhibit their growth.

MICROSCOPY
Light Microscopy

The **brightfield microscope** is used for the majority of routine examinations, especially of stained specimens.

The **darkfield microscope** is a form of light microscope in which an opaque stop is inserted below or into the condenser to allow only peripheral rays of light to pass. The rays pass through the specimen at such an angle that the field appears unilluminated, and the organisms appear bright against a dark background because they reflect the light. This type of microscopy is especially useful in examining microorganisms which are

Table 2-1. Types of Microscopy Useful in the Examination of Bacteria

Microscope	Source	Approximate maximum magnification	Uses
Brightfield	Visible light	1,000×	Examination of routine stained specimens
Darkfield	Visible light	1,000×	Examination of microorganisms difficult to stain; motility studies
Phase-contrast	Visible light	1,000×	Examination of unstained histologic sections
Flourescent	UV light	1,000×	Fluorescent antibody techniques
Transmission electron microscope	Electron beam	200,000×	Examination of subcellular ultrastructure
Scanning electron microscope	Electron beam	10,000×	Examination of surface structures

difficult to stain, e.g., spirochetes. Ordinarily, living organisms in wet-mount preparations are examined with this technique, and therefore it is also useful in studies of motility.

The **phase microscope** utilizes a halo of light produced by light passing from the source through an annular diaphragm. The rays of light passing through areas of varying refractive index emerge out of phase and produce a pattern of bright and dark relief. This form of microscopy is useful in examining bacteria in histologic sections, since the microorganisms are of a different refractive index than the surrounding tissue and consequently are visible without special staining.

Fluorescent Microscopy

The **fluorescent microscope** is used primarily with the fluorescent antibody technique in diagnostic microbiology. Ultraviolet light is employed because it is absorbed by certain fluorescent chemical complexes which then emit rays of visible light. Microorganisms are treated with a fluorescent dye or specific antibody conjugated with fluorescein to make them visible. A variety of bacteria including group A streptococci and enteropathogenic *Escherichia coli* can be identified by means of the fluorescent antibody technique.

Electron Microscopy

Electron microscopy is based upon the use of an electron source instead of a light source, and magnets instead of lenses.

The **transmission electron microscope** allows magnifications up to 200,000×. A finely focused beam of electrons passes through specially prepared ultrathin sections; the beam is then refocused, and the image is essentially a reflection of what the specimen does to the transmitted electron beam. Specimen preparation is difficult and time-consuming, and interpretation requires considerable experience. The major use of transmission electron microscopy is in studying the ultrastructure of microorganisms.

The **scanning electron microscope** allows true magnification of up to only 10,000×, but provides images in three-dimensional perspective. A finely focused beam of electrons scans the specimen like a television raster, and the image is the result of secondary electrons emitted from the surface of the specimen by the incident electron beam. This instrument is specifically useful in studying the surface structure of intact cells. Preparation of specimens is simple because sectioning is not required, and interpretation is relatively easy because the image correlates well with previous visual experience.

The various types of microscopy are demonstrated in Figure 2-1, revealing how one organism appears with each microscopic technique.

STAINING   Bacterial cells contain no chlorophyll and therefore are naturally colorless and transparent. For this reason, and because the bacterial cell is poorly refractile, straining is of primary importance in visualizing bacterial morphology by light microscopy. Although a myriad of routine and special stains are available, only those most commonly used are mentioned.

Gram Stain

Gram stain is the most commonly employed and important of all stains utilized for visualizing bacteria. By this method bacteria are classified into two major groups: those which are gram-positive and those that are gram-negative. Gram-positive bacteria stain deep purple because they retain the primary dye complex (methyl violet and iodine) following attempted decolorization with alcohol-acetone solution. Gram-negative bacteria are decolorized and appear red because they stain with the counter stain (safranin). This staining procedure therefore not only allows visualization of form, size, shape, and other structural details, but allows microorganisms to be artificially grouped by their staining reaction.

Acid-Fast Stains

Another useful differential staining technique is the acid-fast stain, which is most commonly used to identify the tubercle bacillus and other mycobacteria, organisms difficult to stain with ordinary dyes. In the acid-fast technique, basic dyes are employed with heat in the presence of acid. Once stained, mycobacteria are resistant to acid-alcohol, which decolorizes most other bacteria. The Ziehl-Neelsen stain is the most commonly used and employs carbofuchsin as the primary stain and methylene blue as the counterstain to provide contrasting color for ease in viewing. In this system, acid-fast bacteria appear red-purple, and nonacid-fast microorganisms appear blue. Acidfastness is probably a reflection of the selective permeability of the cell membrane. The red color of acid-fast organisms is due to the retention of the carbolfuchsin dye; disruption of the cell results in loss of this staining property.

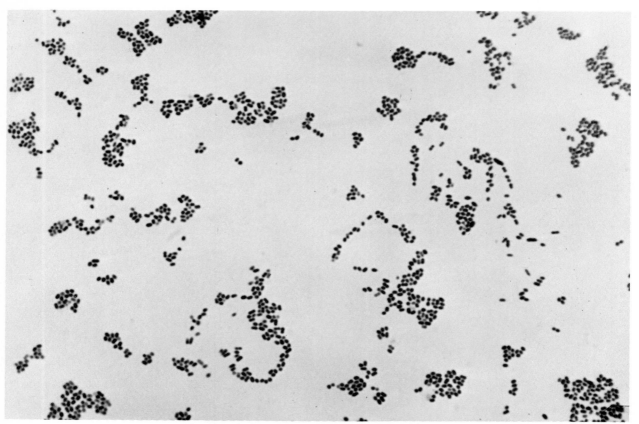

A

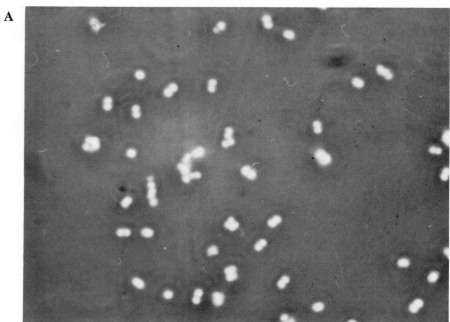

B

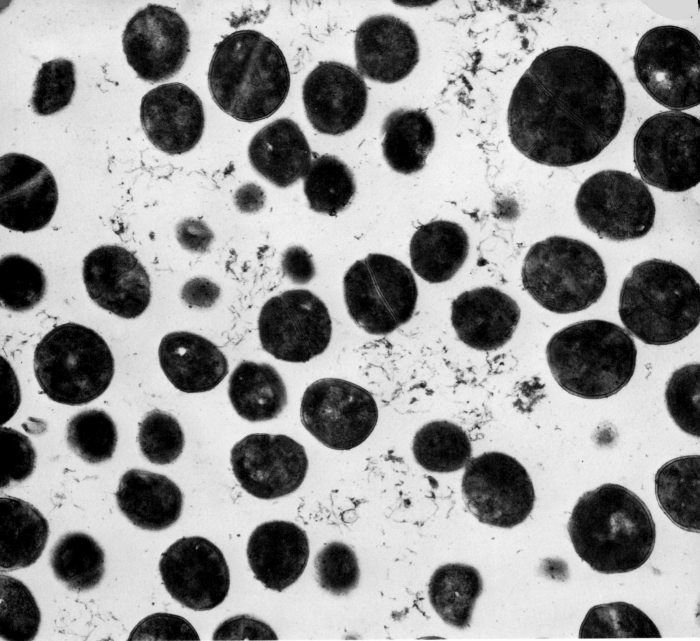

C

Fig. 2–1.
Staphylococcus aureus as visualized with different forms of microscopy.
A. Gram stain visualized by brightfield microscopy.
B. Phase microscopic view.
C. Transmission electron micrograph.
(**A, B,** ×1,000; **C,** ×30,000)
(*Continued*)

(*Fig. 2–1, continued*)
D. Scanning electron micrograph.
(**D**, × 10,000)

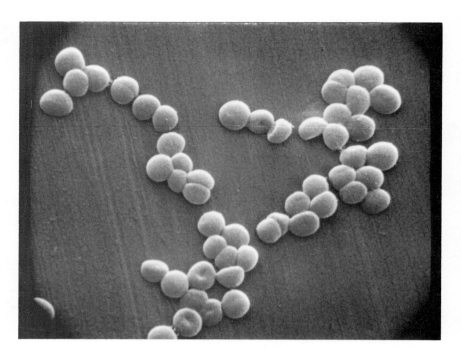

D

India Ink Preparations   Suspensions of microorganisms are mixed with India ink. These preparations are particularly useful for visualizing capsules, especially of cryptococci, and are dependent on the fact that the capsule displaces the colloidal carbon particles of the ink, resulting in a clear halo around the microorganism.

CULTURAL TECHNIQUES   Diagnostic bacteriology is dependent on obtaining pure cultures of bacteria that can be used to study colonial characteristics, the morphology of individual cells, biochemical properties, and staining and immunologic reactions. Excellent descriptions of the various culture techniques have been published and are not included in this text. However, since bacteria in the environment, in the infected host, and in culture media display certain basic properties of nutrition and growth, these and the environmental factors which influence them are summarized.

NUTRITION AND GROWTH
Nutrition   Bacteria are characterized by their nutritional requirements as 1) **saprophytes** (bacteria which consume organic matter derived from dead organisms or their excreta; 2) **parasites** (bacteria which consume organic matter obtained from living organisms; or 3) **autotrophic bacteria** (bacteria for which the principal nutrients are inorganic). Most bacteria which cause human disease are either saprophytes or parasites. The basic nutritional requirements of bacteria are an energy source, a source of carbon, a source of nitrogen for the synthesis of proteins and nucleic acids, and a source of other accessory growth factors such as inorganic salts, vitamins, lipids,

organic acids, amino acids, purines, and pyrimidines. Bacteria vary considerably with regard to the simplicity or complexity of their nutritional requirements, and these differences provide the basis for selective inhibitory media utilized in their isolation and identification.

Environmental factors and the concentration of specific nutrients significantly affect the growth and metabolism of bacteria.

Oxygen. Most bacteria grow under a wide range of oxygen tension, but the oxygen requirement for growth is useful as a further means of classifying broad groups. **Obligate aerobes** grow only if oxygen is available, e.g., the tubercle bacillus. **Obligate anaerobes** require the absence of oxygen in their environment, e.g., the tetanus bacillus; many obligate anaerobes not only grow poorly but die in the presence of oxygen. **Microaerophilic bacteria** grow optimally in the presence of low levels of oxygen. Most bacteria are **facultative anaerobes**, i.e., they grow under a wide range of oxygen tensions and can grow in the presence or absence of air. Bacteria can also be classified by their use of oxygen as electron acceptors. Organisms capable of transferring electrons from organic materials to oxygen are said to respire; those transferring electrons to organic acceptors are said to ferment (the fermentation process is variable and a number of distinctive types are known, e.g., alcoholic, lactic, formic; the enzymes and endproducts of fermentation aid in the identification of many bacteria).

Water. Water makes up more than 80% of the bacterial cell and is essential for growth. Loss of water is tolerated differently by various species. Spores are very resistant to drying and may survive for many years in the desiccated state.

Light. All parasitic bacteria survive best and grow optimally in darkness. Diffuse sunlight is harmful because of the ultraviolet light present in its rays.

Temperature. Temperature is an important variable in determining optimal growth of bacteria. Bacteria can be classified into groups based on their optimum temperature ranges. **Psychrophiles** grow well at low temperatures (20°–30°C). **Thermophiles** grow best at 55°–60° or higher. **Mesophiles** grow optimally at intermediate temperatures (37°–40°C) and represent the most important group of medical interest. For each organism there is an optimum temperature range for growth; this may be different for other cell functions such as respiration and fermentation.

Hydrogen Ion Concentration. Most organisms grow optimally in the neutral range (pH 7.2–7.4), but some are more acid- and/or base-tolerant (the extremes of microbial tolerance are pH are 4 to 10).

Salts. Salts in high concentration are generally toxic; in low concentration they support growth.

Specific Ions. Certain ions, such as magnesium, iron, phosphate, potassium, manganese, cobalt, copper, and calcium, play specific roles; for example, *Corynebacterium diphtheriae* produces toxin only within a very narrow range of iron concentration.

Growth and Cell Division

Under ideal conditions, one bacterium can divide into two bacteria every 15 to 20 minutes. However, as shown above, many factors affect growth and the usual way of defining growth is by the **logarithmic** or **exponential growth curve,** a sigmoidal curve obtained by plotting the log number of organisms growing under specified conditions as a function of time. There are four parts of the growth curve: 1) the lag phase, a period during which there is an increase in cell mass without a significant increase in cell number; 2) the logarithmic or exponential phase (the period during which the rate of increase in cell number remains constant; 3) the stationary or maximum phase (a period during which cells begin to die owing to limitation in nutrients, production of noxious metabolic by-products, etc., and cell count remains stationary); and 4) the decline phase (a period of reduction in the cell count). Specifically with regard to growth, the phase of logarithmic or exponential growth is most important, and certain common definitions are pertinent to it. The exponential phase of growth is a period of balanced growth when every cell component including cell number increases by a constant factor. The more optimum the environment, the faster the cells divide; this is expressed as the mean generation time (MGT) or doubling time, the time in which the number of cells doubles. The MGT is a useful parameter which reflects the ability of the bacteria to grow and divide in a relatively controlled environment. The MGT is affected by nutrition, oxygenation, temperature, and the other factors mentioned above which affect cell growth and metabolism. Most important to remember, however, is that growth in any system is a dynamic process involving a myriad of interactions between the microorganism and its environment.

In general, bacteria reproduce by binary fission. The cell elongates, a transverse cell membrane is formed (Figs. 1-2 and 1-3), and subsequently a new cell wall develops. The new transverse septum and cell wall grow inward from the outer layers. During cell division the nuclear material doubles before division and is distributed equally to the two daughter cells. Bacteria lack a mitotic spindle; the developing transverse septum separates the duplicated chromosomal material. Cell groupings are determined by the plane of division and the number of divisions through which the daughter cells remain attached, as discussed in Chapter 1, *Structure and Morphology of Bacteria.*

SUGGESTED READING

1. CHERRY WB, GOLDMAN M, CARSKI TR, et al: Fluorescent Antibody Techniques in the Diagnosis of Communicable Diseases. Public Health Service Publication No. 729. Washington, DC, Government Printing Office, 1960

2. DAVIS BD, DULBECCO R, EISEN HN, et al: Microbiology. Second edition. Hagerstown, Md, Harper and Row, 1973, pp 39–105

3. RICHARDS OW: Microscopy, Manual of Clinical Microbiology. Edited by JE Blair, EH Lennette, JP Truant. Bethesda, Md, American Society for Microbiology, 1970, pp 13–27

Pathogenesis of Bacterial Disease

Just how bacteria cause disease is not entirely understood, but it is generally agreed that the two most important pathogenetic mechanisms are invasion and destruction of host tissues and the production of toxins.

HOST VERSUS PARASITE
Tissue Invasion

When bacteria invade a host, proliferate, and disseminate, injury to and destruction of host cells and tissues occurs both locally at the site of invasion and also distally if metastatic infection occurs via bacteremic spread. Ordinarily bacteria cause disease by both invasion and toxin production, but some species are pathogenic primarily due to their invasive properties, e.g., pneumococci. In great part the ability of an organism to cause disease by invasion of tissue is determined by its ability to survive the attempts of the host to contain and destroy it; this is related to whether it is an extracellular or intracellular parasite. Extracellular parasites (e.g., *Diplococcus pneumoniae, Streptococcus pyogenes, Staphylococcus aureus*) are capable of producing disease only so long as they remain outside the phagocytic cells of the host; in contrast, intracellular parasites (e.g., *Salmonella typhosa, Brucella abortus*) can survive and multiply within phagocytic cells and may destroy them. The ultimate result of bacterial invasion is due in greater part, however, to the location of the disease process and how critical the involved tissues are to the survival of the host. For example, destruction of a limb may not significantly alter the viability of the host, but a small abscess in a vital area of the midbrain or a septic embolus to a major coronary artery may be incompatible with life.

Toxin Production

Exotoxins are heat-labile toxic proteins produced within certain gram-positive and a few gram-negative bacterial cells; they are released into the surrounding medium without appreciable damage to the cell itself. The principal bacterial exotoxins which cause disease in man are listed in Table 3-1. Exposure of exotoxins to heat, formaldehyde, and other denaturing agents results in a decrease in toxicity but does not alter antigenicity. Toxins treated in such a manner are called **toxoids;** some (e.g., tetanus and diphtheria toxoids) are widely used to induce active immunity.

Endotoxins are relatively heat-stable (do not form toxoids), complex macromolecules containing both phospholipid and polysaccharide; they are an integral part of the cell wall of gram-negative bacteria and are released only if cellular integrity is altered. The toxicity of an endotoxin resides in the phospholipid fraction, and its specific antigenicity in the polysaccharide moiety. The biologic actions of endotoxins are many, but their ultimate mechanism of action in causing disease has not been entirely elucidated. In man, endotoxin induces the clinical picture of shock (gram-negative shock, endotoxin shock).

Endotoxin shock is a dynamic syndrome that is the result of infection by gram-negative bacteria and release of endotoxin, causing inadequate perfusion of blood into the tissues. Although the microcirculation of the capillary loop is the final determinant of the events that occur in endotoxin shock, multiple factors are involved in the genesis and persistence of the progressive decompensation of the capillary circulation and the cells that it supports. Gram-negative bacteremia is common but not a prerequisite for the development of endotoxin shock; all that is necessary is the release of endotoxin. This condition is essentially a disease of hospitalized patients and is second only to myocardial infarction as a cause of death on many large medical services. It is most common in men over 40 years of age but is fairly frequent in women with septic abortions. Among the factors predisposing to the infections with which this syndrome is associated are urinary, intestinal, biliary tract, or gynecologic manipulations or surgery; transfusion of contaminated blood; hepatic cirrhosis; diabetes mellitus; burns; cancer (especially of the hematopoietic system); and the use of radiotherapy, antimetabolites, corticosteroids, and antibiotics. The organisms most often involved are *Escherichia coli, Proteus* species, *Pseudomonas aeruginosa,* and bacteroides. Hypotension is present in about 80% of patients who have gram-negative bacteremia, but only about 20% develop the syndrome of shock; the fatality rate in the latter group is 40–80% and has remained unchanged even in recent years, making endotoxin shock one of the most life-threatening clinical entities seen in hospitalized patients.

Table 3-1. Principal Bacterial Exotoxins Which Cause Disease in Man

Toxigenic species	Toxin	Disease
Clostridium botulinum	Type-specific neu-rotoxins	Botulism
Clostridium perfringens	α-Toxins and others	Gas gangrene
Clostridium tetani	Tetanospasmin; tetanolysin	Tetanus
Corynebacterium diphtheriae	Diphtheria toxin	Diphtheria
Staphylococcus aureus	α-, β-, γ-toxins; leukocidin	Staphylococcal pyogenic infections
	Enterotoxin	Staphylococcal food poisoning
	Erythrogenic toxin	Staphylococcal scarlet fever
Streptococcus pyogenes	Streptolysins O and S	Streptococcal pyogenic infections
	Erythrogenic toxin	Streptococcal scarlet fever

BACTERIAL DISEASES   Disease caused by bacteria is basically the end result of the conflict between invading bacteria and the host. If the former are the victors, disease occurs; if the latter, the bacteria are contained, destroyed, and usually eliminated from the body. Both the bacteria and the host have certain inherent defense mechanisms which play a significant role in determining this outcome.

Bacterial Defense Mechanisms   The capsules of certain extracellular parasites are antiphagocytic and protect the organism from being ingested by the phagocytes of the host. Such antiphagocytic capsules contribute significantly to the virulence of certain species such as *Diplococcus pneumoniae*. Antibody to the capsular polysaccharide of such organisms destroys this antiphagocytic property. Spore formation is probably another defense mechanism. Certain properties of bacteria, such as their ability to elaborate extracellular enzymes, contribute to their invasiveness, but whether these are specifically protective is uncertain.

Host Defense Mechanisms   *Normal Indigenous Flora.* The normal exogenous and endogenous micro-flora in the host provide a unique system of checks and balances; they result in a symbiotic state qualitatively and quantitatively dependent upon a stable though dynamic microbial population.

Anatomic Barriers and Secretions. The skin and mucous membranes act as barriers between the internal and external environments of the host. Further protective value is related to their anatomic characteristics, such as the trapping effect of the mucus-coated hairs in the nose and the expulsive action of the cilia of the upper respiratory tract. The antimicrobial nature of their secretions also plays a role. Gastric hydrochloric acid, for example, has a profound antibacterial effect on many microorganisms; unsaturated fatty acids in skin protect against dermal infection; and secretory immunoglobulins in the upper respiratory and gastrointestinal tracts undoubtedly play a significant role in defense against infection.

Inflammation and Phagocytosis. The local inflammatory response to the presence of microorganisms in the tissues is mediated by both local and systemic factors which work in concert to localize and contain the infectious process. Early there is a vascular response mediated by histamine and the kinins as well as other less well characterized biologically active mediators. These cause constriction of the pre- and postcapillary sphincters followed by capillary dilatation and increased capillary permeability. Simultaneously there is adherence of phagocytic cells to the capillary endothelium and subsequent migration of phagocytes through the widened intercellular spaces into the area of bacterial infection; there they phagocytize bacteria with the aid of antibody. (Phagocytosis is enhanced by the presence of antibodies called **opsonins,** which coat the surface of bacteria and facilitate their ingestion by the phagocyte.) The movement of phagocytes within the area of inflammation is affected by **chemotaxins,** substances which attract leukocytes, direct their movement, and thus enhance contact between bacteria and phagocytes. The early inflammatory cell population is composed largely of neutrophils, but these are followed by mononuclear phagocytes, which in turn ingest necrotic tissue debris, bacteria, and dead neutrophils. Mononuclear phagocytes also play a role in transferring antigens from the invading microorganism to lymphocytes in order to stimulate the synthesis of specific antibody.

Phagocytosis is the process of ingestion of a foreign particle by a phagocytic cell. Phagocytic cells are generally of three types: 1) neutrophils, 2) wandering macrophages, i.e., monocytes, and 3) fixed macrophages, i.e., the cells of the reticuloendothelial (RE) system, which is composed of Kupffer cells of the liver, littoral cells of the spleen, reticular cells of lymph nodes, dust cells of the lung, and certain cells in the bone marrow, adrenal glands, pituitary, kidneys, and loose connective tissue. Phagocytosis is composed of three stages: 1) attachment of the cell membrane of the phagocyte to the particle to be ingested, 2) ingestion, and 3) intracellular lysis (Fig. 3-1). In some way—probably related to chance contact, the relative number of phagocytes and particles, and the electrical charge and geometry of the system with enchancement by chemotaxins—the cell membrane of the phagocyte attaches to bacteria either by pseudopod formation (Figs. 3-2 and 3-3) or by trapping the microorganism between the cell membrane of the phagocyte and a random surface (Figs. 3-4 and 3-5). Ingestion is basically engulfment of bacteria by changes in the gel-sol state of the cell membrane of the phagocyte (Fig. 3-1). The bacteria become surrounded by a membrane-lined vacuole (Fig. 3-6) containing lysosomes, membrane-enclosed collections of lytic enzymes capable of destroying some bacteria; these include lysozyme (Fig. 3-7), alkaline phosphatase, acid phosphatase, ribonuclease, deoxyribonuclease, β-glucuronidase, and nucleotidase. When these enzymes are released the ingested bacteria are lysed; it should be emphasized, though, that phagocytosis does not ensure intracellular killing; in some cases, the engulfed microorganism may survive and even multiply within phagocytes. Nevertheless, the inflamma-

Fig. 3–1.
The process of phagocytosis by human polymorphonuclear leukocytes.

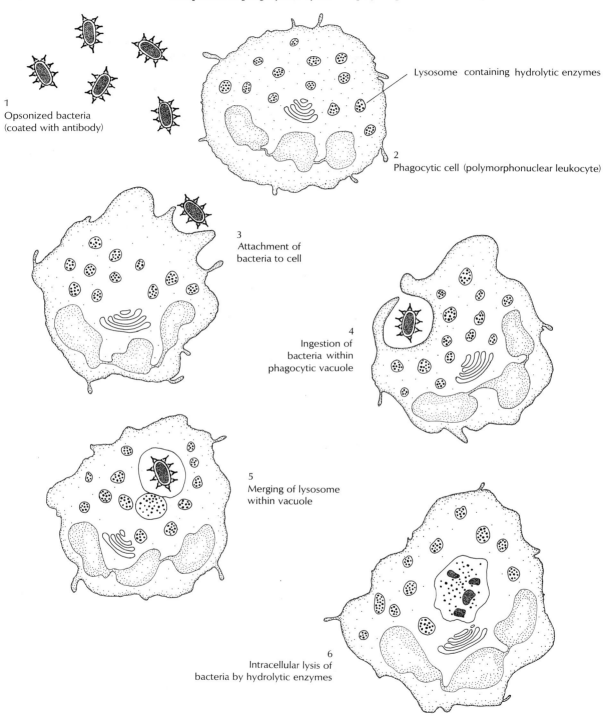

1
Opsonized bacteria
(coated with antibody)

Lysosome containing hydrolytic enzymes

2
Phagocytic cell (polymorphonuclear leukocyte)

3
Attachment of
bacteria to cell

4
Ingestion of
bacteria within
phagocytic vacuole

5
Merging of lysosome
within vacuole

6
Intracellular lysis of
bacteria by hydrolytic enzymes

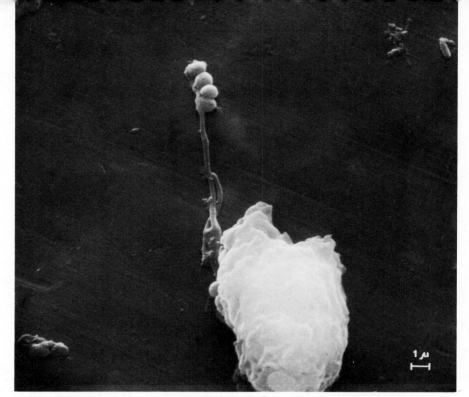

Fig. 3–2.
Scanning electron micrograph of a single pseudopod of a human polymorphonuclear leukocyte in suspension attaching to each of a group of four staphylococci. (×5,000)

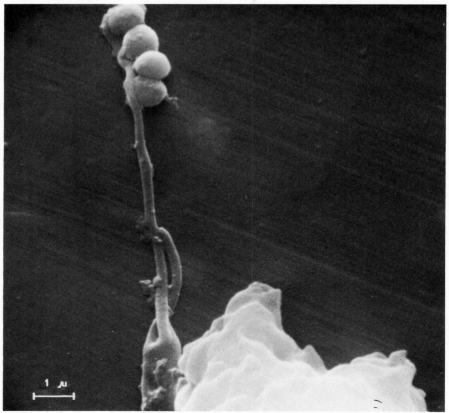

Fig. 3–3.
Magnified view of Figure 3–2, demonstrating the attachment of a pseudopod of a polymorphonuclear leukocyte to each of four staphylococci. (×10,000)

Fig. 3–4.
Scanning electron micrograph of a human polymorphonuclear leukocyte on glass, illustrating the fern-like nature of the cell membrane of the phagocyte on a glass surface. (×5,000)

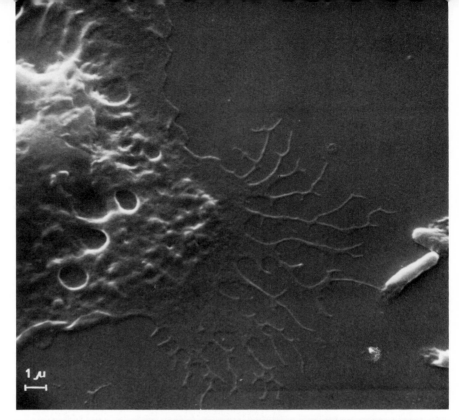

Fig. 3–5.
Scanning electron micrograph of a human polymorphonuclear leukocyte in suspension trapping *Proteus mirabilis* between its membrane and the surface (surface phagocytosis). (×5,000)

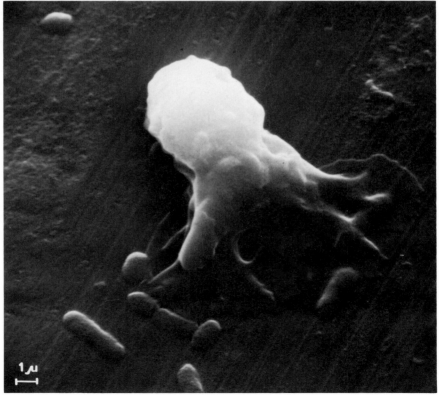

Fig. 3–6.
Human polymorphonuclear leukocyte on glass, demonstrating phagocytic vacuoles. Staphylococci can be seen attached to the periphery of the phagocyte and within the vacuoles. (×5,000)

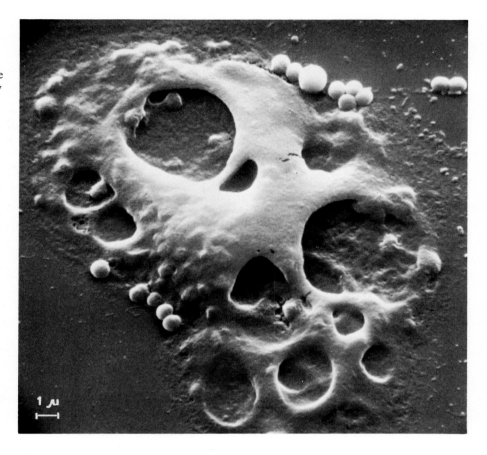

Table 3-2. Common Types of Antibodies

Type of antibody	Reaction of antigen
Antitoxins	Neutralize or flocculate toxins or toxoids
Agglutinins	Immobilize motile organisms or cause aggregation of cells or particles to form chunks; agglutinins can be demonstrated only if the antigen is particulate or absorbed onto the surface of a particle, e.g., an erythrocyte or a latex particle
Precipitins	Form complexes with antigen in solution resulting in precipitation; precipitins can be demonstrated only if the antigen is soluble
Lysins	Lyse antigenic cells, usually in the presence of complement
Opsonins	Combine with surface components of bacteria or other cells to enhance ingestion by phagocytes
Neutralizing (protective)	Protect the host by neutralizing the effects of the antigenic micro-organism
Complement-fixing	Participate in antigen-antibody reactions which consume or "fix" complement
Blocking	Combine with specific antigen, but are detected by demonstration that they block another reaction

tory response, the process of phagocytosis, and the RE system with its effective and efficient filtration network inherent in the sinusoidal architecture of the lymph nodes, liver, and spleen provide a unique system for clearing microorganisms and protecting the host against the dissemination of infection.

Immune System, Antibody, and Complement. **Antibody** may be defined as an immunoglobulin of specific structure synthesized in response to a specific antigen. (An **antigen** is a substance which elicits the formation of antibody.) The mechanism whereby anibodies are formed in response to antigen is still uncertain, but an acceptable simple hypothesis is diagramed in Figure 3-8. The common types of antibodies are noted in Table 3-2.

The common types of host immunity are as follows:

1. **Active immunity:** Immunity acquired by effective exposure to a microorganism or its products. It develops slowly over a period of days or weeks and generally persists for years; it is acquired principally by exposure to the natural disease (clinical or subclinical) or by the use of the many immunizations currently available.

2. **Passive immunity:** A state of relative temporary immunity induced by the administration of antibody formed in another host rather than actively formed by the individual. Protection lasts only a short time (usually less than 4 weeks, since this preformed antibody is breaking down without the synthesis of new antibody), but protection is immediate since there is no lag period required for the formation of active immunity. Examples of passive immunity are the administration of hyperimmune gamma globulin or antitoxins, and the transfer of maternal antibody to the fetus.

3. **Natural immunity:** Immunity not acquired by previous known contact with specific antigen or the administration of preformed antibody (active and passive immunity are acquired), but inherent in a host. This includes the immunity to infection observed in certain species (species immunity), races (racial or genetic immunity), or individuals (individual resistance). An example of natural immunity is the inherent immunity of the dark-skinned races to falciparum malaria.

The **immunoglobulins** are plasma proteins synthesized by lymphoid and plasma cells. Their subunits—the heavy chains and light chains—are structurally similar; differences in the former provide the basis for the five commonly recognized classes: IgG, IgM, IgA, IgE, and IgD. Although the term immunoglobulin implies that these substances are antibodies, not all immunoglobulins are; IgD has no known immunobiologic function. The other four immunoglobulins are antibodies and play variable roles in the immune component of the overall host defense system.

IgM is the largest of the immunoglobulins, having a molecular weight of 900,000. IgM is usually the first immunoglobulin to appear in response to an antigenic stimulus; this is followed by a rise in IgG which, via a feedback mechanism, inhibits the synthesis of IgM.

IgG has a molecular weight of 150,000 and is the most plentiful of the immunoglobulins. It is present at birth, being contributed by the mother;

Fig. 3–7.
Lysozyme: molecular structure and substrate.
A. Lysozyme molecule without the substrate. Shown in outline are the four disulfide bridges that help maintain the three-dimensional conformation of this enzyme. The crevice across the molecule into which the substrate fits is indicated by a dashed line.

A

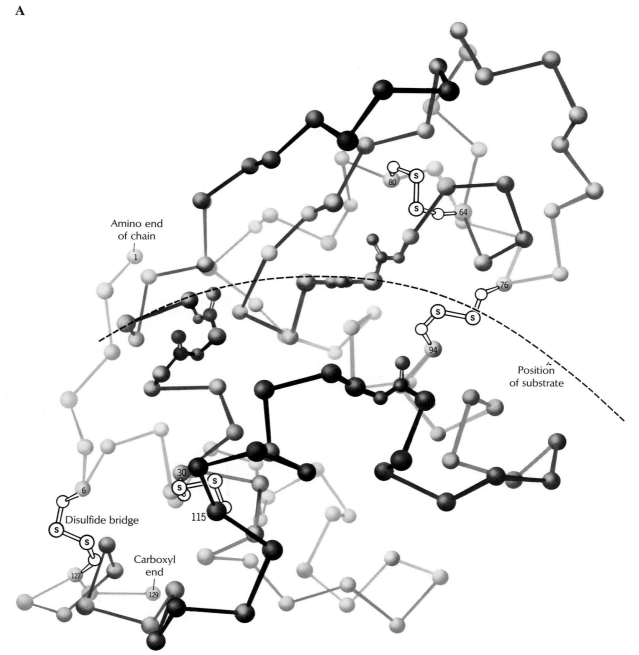

B. Lysozyme with the hexasaccharide substrate in position. The substrate upon which lysozyme acts is part of the cell wall of bacteria (see **C**). The main chain of the substrate is shown by the heavy black lines. (Substrate side chains are gray.) The side chains of the molecule that interact with the substrate are shown in outline. Rings *A*, *B*, and *C* come from observed trimer binding. Rings *D*, *E*, and *F* are inferred from model building. (**A** and **B** adapted from p71 of Dickerson RE, Geis I: The Structure and Action of Proteins. Menlo Park, Calif, WA Benjamin, 1969)
(*Continued*)

B

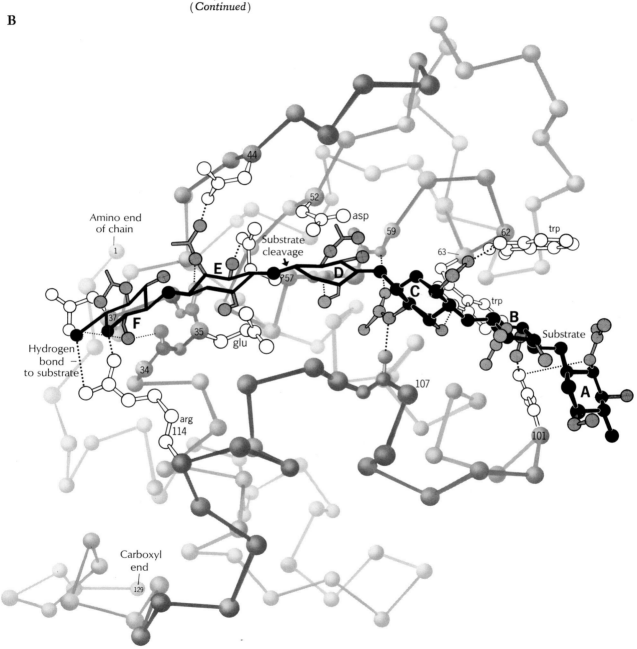

(*Fig. 3–7, continued*)

C. The substrate of lysozyme is an alternating copolymer of N-acetylglucosamine (NAG) and N-acetylmuramic acid (NAM) units or part of the bacterial cell wall. Shown here is the detailed binding of the substrate to the molecule. (**C**, Dickerson RE, Geis I: The Structure and Action of Proteins. Menlo Park, Calif, WA Benjamin, 1969)

the levels of IgG then decrease until about the fourth month of life when the child begins to synthesize IgG at a rate greater than its utilization; the levels then remain dynamically stable during life but decrease with old age. IgG synthesis and a rise in serum levels follows that of IgM after primary immunization, but IgG is the major immunoglobulin reflecting the anamnestic response.

IgA (secretory immunoglobulin) is present principally in mucous epithelial surfaces, such as the nasal, bronchial, and intestinal mucosa. Its primary function is to protect the mucous membranes against invasion and infection by microorganisms.

IgE is present in serum in only very small amounts. IgE antibodies affix themselves to the skin and other cells and may be important in the protection of the respiratory tract against infection.

The complement system is a group of plasma proteins which play an important role in the overall system of host defenses. The **complement cascade** consists of nine components acting in sequence (Fig. 3-9). The various components of complement participate in immune adherence, chemotaxis, phagocytosis, intracellular killing of phagocytized bacteria, and release of vasoactive mediators.

Whereas the immunoglobulins represent humoral or circulating antibody which can be transferred by serum, **delayed hypersensitivity** reflects cell-bound antibody. Delayed hypersensitivity reactions develop more slowly, persist longer, and cannot be transferred by serum. The prototype of the delayed hypersensitivity reaction is tuberculin sensitivity.

The immune response is a complex integrated system which plays a major role in protecting the host against infection, but it should be remembered that detectable antibody is not demonstrable until 5 to 7 days after the first exposure to antigens. Most infections are "first" infections, and therefore the immune response is of little immediate value; it is of far greater importance in the previously sensitized host in whom the anamnestic response endows his immunity with specific immediate value.

TRANSMISSION OF BACTERIAL INFECTIONS

In order to infect, bacteria must be transmitted to a host in some way. The common modes of transmission are as follows:

1. Direct transmission (man to man)
   a. Contact with secretions from an infected person via sneezing, coughing, speaking, breathing
   b. Transmission from the mother to the fetus via the placenta
2. Indirect transmission
   a. Via food, milk, water
   b. Via fomites
   c. Via infected droplets in air
   d. Via dust
   e. Via arthropod vectors

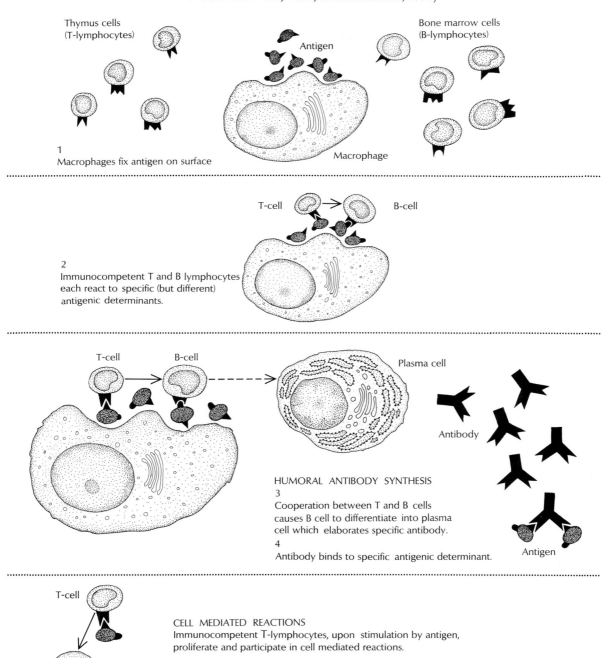

Fig. 3–8.
Theoretical concept of the immune response, including antibody formation and cell-mediated reactions. (Adapted from Immunobiology. Edited by RA Good and DW Fisher. Stamford, Conn, Sinauer Associate, 1971)

Thymus cells
(T-lymphocytes)

Antigen

Bone marrow cells
(B-lymphocytes)

1
Macrophages fix antigen on surface

Macrophage

T-cell   B-cell

2
Immunocompetent T and B lymphocytes each react to specific (but different) antigenic determinants.

T-cell   B-cell   Plasma cell

Antibody

HUMORAL ANTIBODY SYNTHESIS
3
Cooperation between T and B cells causes B cell to differentiate into plasma cell which elaborates specific antibody.
4
Antibody binds to specific antigenic determinant.

Antigen

T-cell

CELL MEDIATED REACTIONS
Immunocompetent T-lymphocytes, upon stimulation by antigen, proliferate and participate in cell mediated reactions.

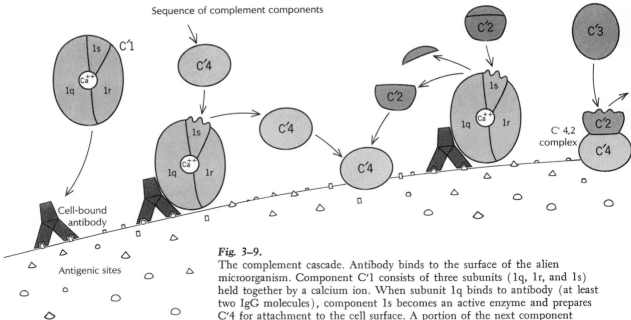

Sequence of complement components

Cell-bound antibody

Antigenic sites

C' 4,2 complex

Fig. 3–9.

The complement cascade. Antibody binds to the surface of the alien microorganism. Component C'1 consists of three subunits (1q, 1r, and 1s) held together by a calcium ion. When subunit 1q binds to antibody (at least two IgG molecules), component 1s becomes an active enzyme and prepares C'4 for attachment to the cell surface. A portion of the next component C'2 is split off to enable it to join C'4. C'4,2 complex can now act as an amplifier and activate numbers of C'3 molecules for binding to the cell surface. Components C'5, C'6, and C'7, either separately or as a unit, bind to the cell surface. C'8 component binds to the cell, after which C'9 binds to C'8 and induces the C'8 molecule to produce holes in the cell membrane. This results in destruction of the alien cell (erythrocyte or bacterium) by lysis. [Note: $\overline{C4,2}$ is now the preferred convention for indicating the complement cascade. It replaces the C'4,2 notation used here.] (Illustration from Dickerson RE, Geis I: The Structure and Action of Proteins. Menlo Park, Calif, WA Benjamin, 1969)

For effective transmission to occur there must be a source of the infecting agent, i.e., a significant number of microorganisms capable of surviving the medium of transmission. In addition, the potential host must be susceptible, although even immune persons may carry and disseminate a microorganism without suffering the disease which the bacteria produce in the nonimmune individual.

OPPORTUNISTIC INFECTION   Under normal circumstances man lives in delicate and dynamic balance with the microorganisms of his internal and external environments. Infectious disease occurs when pathogenic organisms upset this balance and penetrate a sequence of defensive barriers, proliferate, and disseminate throughout the infected host. In distinct contrast, infection by the varied but characteristic microorganisms that constitute the normal indigenous flora rarely occurs in the healthy host. Disease due to the ubiquitous, saprophytic, "nonpathogenic," or "nonvirulent" commensals is designated **opportunistic infection,** a term which also implies some derangement in host defense mechanisms so as to provide the opportunity for infection to

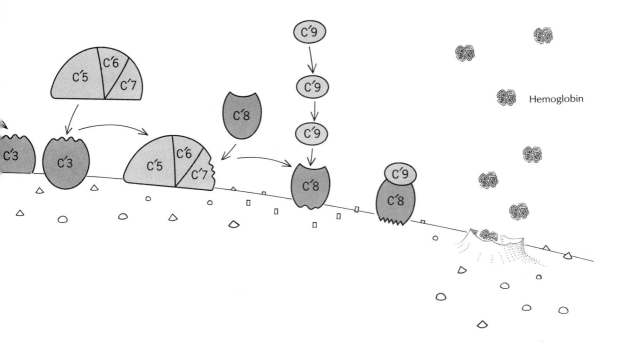

Hemoglobin

begin. Although the basic concepts of infectious diseases due to either pathogenic or nonpathogenic microorganisms are similar, the term opportunistic infection is used to designate only those infections caused by organisms not generally regarded as pathogenic.

Once considered rare, opportunistic infections represent an increasingly important chapter in the study and management of infectious diseases. Man-to-man, insect vector, and filth-borne transmission maintain their primary positions in the spread of recognized pathogens and have been brought under some degree of control. In contrast, diseases due to indigenous and saprophytic microorganisms are being seen with increasing frequency, especially in medical centers where complex diagnostic, operative, and therapeutic procedures are employed. Advances in medical science have created a growing population whose survival, though prolonged by modern medicine, is constantly threatened by opportunistic infection. We are now able to prolong the lives of persons with severe and debilitating underlying disease; we have acquired a new armamentarium of diagnostic techniques and therapeutic agents; and we have taken significant steps into the era of transplantation and implantation of natural and synthetic tissues and organs. Infection, more than any other single factor, has hindered our success in these areas, and the opportunistic microorganisms have emerged as major pathogens.

Host Factors   Infection by opportunistic microorganisms usually results from a deficiency in host defense mechanisms rather than from the *de novo* acquisition of increased virulence by these microorganisms. The role of

Pathogenesis of Bacterial Disease   **49**

Table 3-3. Normal and Altered Host Defenses in Opportunistic Infection

Normal host defense	Predisposing factors	Possible mechanism
Protection afforded by normal flora	Burns, trauma, other infection	May alter normal skin flora by changing skin ecology and physiochemical properties
	Surgery	Preoperative or prophylactic antibiotics may alter normal flora
	Hospitalization	May colonize host with new or resistant organisms
	Antibiotics	See Table 3-4
Anatomic barriers and secretions	Burns, trauma, surgery, other infection, inflammatory diseases	See above; also direct penetration or other disruption of integrity provide new portals of entry for microorganisms
	Extremes of age	May alter physiologic defenses, e.g., loss of gastric acidity as a protective mechanism against ingested organisms or toxins; depressed cough reflex, deficient ciliary action in respiratory tract, and defective clearing mechanism in lung predispose to pulmonary infection
	Foreign bodies, prostheses	May act as nidus for infection, provide new portals of entry, or cause obstruction with stasis and infection
	Diagnostic procedures	May provide new portals of entry for microorganisms
	Urinary tract and intravenous catheters	May provide new portals of entry; may result in obstruction, stasis; or may act as nidus for infection
	Antimetabolites, irradiation	See Table 3-5
	Local ischemia	May alter permeability of skin or mucous membranes to produce new portals of entry
Inflammatory response	Diabetes mellitus, renal failure	Accompanying acidosis results in sluggish polymorphonuclear leukocytic response of reduced intensity, defective leukocyte function, ineffective phagocytosis, and lack of fibroblastic proliferation
	Diseases of hematopoietic system	Infiltration of bone marrow may result in deficient and defective granulocytic pool
	Antimetabolites, irradiation, corticosteroids, other drugs	See Table 3-4
Reticuloendothelial (RE) system	Diseases involving the lymphoid or RE systems, e.g., lymphoma, reticulum cell sarcoma	Depress RE system function
	Antimetabolites, x-irradiation, corticosteroids	See Table 3-4

(*Continued*)

Normal host defense	Predisposing factors	Possible mechanism
Immune response	Disease of the lymphoid tissues and RES, e.g., multiple myeloma, chronic lymphatic leukemia	Decrease in normal immunoglobulins, delayed and defective antibody response to antigenic stimuli, and/or production of varying amounts of abnormal immunoglobulins
	Hodgkin's disease	Depression of delayed hypersensitivity early, lymphopenia later
	Dysproteinemias	Nature of defect reflects factor(s) which are lacking
	Extremes of age	During first 3–6 months dependent on maternal antibody; possible decrease in immune response in the elderly
	Debilitating diseases, e.g., liver disease, renal failure	May affect immunity via defects in protein synthesis and cell division
	Antimetabolites, irradiation, corticosteroids	See Table 3-4.

normal and abnormal host defenses in the pathogenesis of opportunistic infection is summarized in Table 3-3.

Infection due to the opportunists generally does not occur in a haphazard fashion but tends to follow certain specific alterations in host defense in an almost predictable manner. Opportunistic infection is not the inevitable consequence of overwhelming disease or the agonal state as evidenced by its rarity in terminal illness due to myocardial infarction, rheumatic heart disease, or cerebrovascular occlusion. In contrast, these infections are not uncommon in persons with leukemia, multiple myeloma, or Hodgkin's disease. This difference in the incidence of opportunistic infection can usually be related to some specific derangement of the host's defenses in each of the latter diseases. To understand the pathogenesis of opportunistic infection fully, therefore, factors which may alter each component of the host defense system must be considered.

Alterations in Anatomic Barriers and Mucous Membranes. Loss of the integrity of the skin or mucous membranes allows entry of a variety of exogenous and endogenous microorganisms. Such loss may be due to trauma or to primary diseases of the skin and mucous membranes as exemplified by the increased incidence of infection in areas of burns or ischemia and by the role of bacteria and bacterial toxins in the morbidity and mortality of intestinal infarction or obstruction. The presence of a foreign body in the bloodstream, tissues, or body cavities predisposes to infection. Cardiac valve replacements, vascular prostheses, and prolonged urinary tract or intravenous catheterization provide foci for chronic infection with saprophytic microorganisms indigenous to specific localities. Local infection can predispose to further problems by injury to mechanical barriers or by other alterations in local defense mechanisms. A current problem of increasing proportion is bacteremia initiated by infection around intravenous catheters, administration of contaminated intravenous solutions, or the self-administration of drugs with nonsterile implements. If this occurs in the presence of defective host defenses or other predisposing factors, life-threatening blood-borne infection, rather than transient bacteremia, may result.

Systemic Factors and Underlying Debilitating Diseases. Conditions such as diabetic acidosis, renal failure, and hepatic failure are complicated frequently by opportunistic infection. Such illnesses are characterized by serious underlying derangements in metabolic balance. However, no single mechanism has been identified as yet to explain the increased susceptibility to infection in these disorders. In patients with acute or chronic renal failure, uremic acidosis contributes to a defect in the early phase of the acute inflammatory response. In addition, uremia results in suppression of the immune response to antigenic stimuli, impaired delayed cutaneous hypersensitivity, and an abnormal production of all classes of immunoglobulins. The uremic patient, as well as those with chronic liver disease, displays defective protein synthesis and cell division. While increased blood sugar *per se* does not play a significant role in altering the severity of systemic infection in the uncontrolled diabetic, the inflammatory response is delayed and defective because of a sluggish polymorphonuclear leukocytic response, ineffective phagocytosis, and a lack of fibroblastic proliferation. Local and systemic metabolic acidosis contributes to this defect. Persons with uncomplicated diabetes do not absorb intramuscularly administered drugs in a normal manner, a factor which may delay effects of therapy. Attempts have been made to analyze the relationships between infectious illness and malnutrition or specific deficiency states. In humans, minimal nutritional deficiency may have no detectable influence on the severity of an infection, whereas moderate to severe nutritional deficiencies may render it more serious. Infection (including "nonspecific diarrhea") is the leading cause of death in children with kwashiorkor. Opportunistic organisms have produced disease in experimental animals with induced deficiencies of vitamin A, niacin, or potassium. In general, however, much information is lacking about the relationship between nutritional states and opportunistic infection.

Disorders Involving the Lymphoid or Reticuloendothelial System. Disorders involving the lymphoid or RE system may result in defective host defense by three major mechanisms: 1) infiltration of the bone marrow by neoplastic cells resulting in an insufficient and defective granulocytic pool; 2) infiltration of the RE system resulting in suppressed function; and 3) changes in serum proteins and antibody formation. Acute leukemia may be characterized by leukopenia with a decrease in the number of polymorphonuclear leukocytes in the peripheral blood and an insufficient granulocytic pool. The majority of patients with acute leukemia have diminished reticuloendothelial phagocytosis except for a few in whom it is increased in relation to accelerated erythrocyte destruction. In contrast, in patients with chronic lymphatic leukemia and multiple myeloma the absolute number of granulocytes is normal or only slightly decreased with normal granulocytic response and phagocytic activity; there is, however, a slowly progressive decrease in normal gamma globulin, defective and delayed antibody response to antigenic stimuli, and production of varying amounts of abnormal serum globulins, which may be related to impaired immunity. There is some evidence that the neoplastic lymphocyte in chronic lymphatic leukemia is immunologically indolent and may fail to play its role in the production of 19S immunoglobulins, thereby jeopardizing protection of the host against gram-negative infections. The immunologic defect in early Hodgkin's disease is characterized by depression of delayed hypersensitivity; antibody formation is essentially normal, and the lymphocyte count is normal or only slightly decreased. Later in the course of the disease there is profound lymphopenia, which probably contributes to the more severe and complex immunologic defects and infectious complications of advanced Hodgkin's disease.

Other Malignancies. Other malignancies, by nature of their size and/or location, may cause obstruction, stasis, ulceration, or hemorrhage; all favor the invasion, growth, and spread of infectious agents.

Dysproteinemias. The dysproteinemias predispose the host to infection, the nature of which is determined by the factors that are absent or present in ineffective quantities.

Age. The very young and the very old display an increased susceptibility to infection. In the former, part of the problem results from lack of protective antibody from the mother until autogenous antibody formation takes place; in the latter, underlying disease, especially congestive heart failure, liver disease, renal disease, and diabetes mellitus, may predispose to infection, as may serum protein changes demonstrable with increasing age.

Therapy   Opportunistic infection has become a major problem primarily since the availability and widespread use of x-irradiation, antimetabolites, antimicrobial agents, and corticosteroids. The roles of various therapeutic efforts leading to an increased incidence of opportunistic infection are outlined in Table 3-4.

The various immunosuppressive and cytotoxic drugs, as well as x-ray therapy, depress the bone marrow and RE system. In addition, cytotoxic drugs injure rapidly growing cells, such as those of the intestinal mucosa, to create new portals of entry for opportunists.

Antibiotics predispose to infection with opportunistic fungi by suppressing the normal bacterial flora of the skin, mucous membranes, and gastrointestinal tract. Antimicrobial agents also alter tissue pH and induce vitamin deficiencies. Chlortetracycline, bacitracin, and neomycin can stimulate the growth and increase the virulence of *Candida albicans*.

Table 3-4. Therapy and Opportunistic Infection

Irradiation and antimetabolites
  Depression of bone marrow with reduced granulocyte and macrophage production
  Suppression of the RE system
  Depression of antibody formation in part by inhibiting the induction phase of the
    immune response and by reducing the mass of antibody forming tissue
  Injury to rapidly growing cells, e.g., mucosa of gastrointestinal tract, producing ulcera-
    tion, bleeding, and subsequent portals of entry for opportunists
Antibiotics
  Alterations in normal microbial flora of skin, mucous membranes, respiratory and
    gastrointestinal tracts
  Selection of resistant species
  Encourage growth of some fungi
Corticosteroids
  Suppression of the inflammatory response
    Delay the onset and decrease the intensity and duration of endothelial sticking of
      leukocytes
    Depress phagocytosis
    Depress intracellular digestion of microorganisms, possibly via stabilization of
      lysosomal membranes
    Depress fibroblastic proliferation
  Depression of antibody formation
    Lympholytic reduction in lymphoid tissue mass
    Depress RE system function
  Suppression of the formation and activity of interferon
Foreign material
  When employed in therapy, may provide route of entry or nidus for microorganisms,
    especially
    Prolonged catheterization of blood vessels, genitourinary tract, etc.
    Vascular, cardiac, or other prosthetic devices
    Sutures
Miscellaneous
  Phenylbutazone may alter phagocytosis
  Dermal preparations and/or allergic reactions to drugs may alter normal microbial
    flora, local secretions, or host surface characteristics to permit invasion by oppor-
    tunists
  Agranulocytosis may complicate drug therapy

Antibiotics cause selective depression of susceptible organisms and result in saprophytic proliferation and selection of resistant species.

Corticosteroid therapy is associated with an increased incidence of infection by opportunistic bacteria, viruses, fungi, and parasites. Pharmacologic amounts of potent glucocorticoid hormones depress all phases of the inflammatory response. A glucocorticoid-induced decrease in antibody synthesis accompanies lysis of lymphoid cells. Large doses depress fibroblastic proliferation and impair RE system activity. Some corticosteroids stabilize lysosomal membranes and thus interfere with release of bacteriolytic enzymes by phagocytes. In addition, adrenocortical hormones in high doses suppress the formation and activity of interferon, a factor of possible importance in opportunistic viral infections.

Table 3-5. *Association of Specific Opportunistic Infections with Certain Predisposing Factors*

Predisposing factor	Frequent opportunistic invaders
Burns, trauma	Pseudomonas and other gram-negative bacilli, staphylococci
Abdominopelvic surgery	Anaerobic streptococci, bacteroides, serratia-enterobacter-klebsiella, straphylococci
Cardiac surgery	Serratia-enterobacter-klebsiella, staphylococci, candida
Intravenous catheters	Staphylococci, aspergilli, candida
Urinary tract manipulation	Proteus, pseudomonas, serratia-enterobacter-klebsiella, staphylococci
Ventriculoatriostomy	Bacilli, staphylococci
Diabetes	Gram-negative bacilli, staphylococci, candida, mucor (with acidosis)
Renal failure	Bacilli, bacteroides, serratia-enterobacter-klebsiella, staphylococci, mucor (with acidosis)
Liver failure	Clostridia, gram-negative bacilli, staphylococci
Diseases involving hemotopoietic, RE, or lymphoid system	Diphtheroids, listeria, pseudomonas and other gram-negative bacilli, staphylococci, nocardia, aspergilli, candida, cryptococci, mucor, cytomegalovirus, herpes zoster, pneumocystis

Microorganisms Causing Opportunistic Infection

That certain disease states are associated with an increased incidence of infection with specific pathogens has been appreciated for some time. The occurrences of salmonella infection in patients with sickle cell disease, streptococcal or staphylococcal infection in patients with cardiovascular disease, and pneumococcal peritonitis in patients with the nephrotic syndrome and cirrhosis are examples of this association. In a similar manner, opportunistic infections occur with relatively predictable associations between specific deficiencies in host defense and an often characteristic etiologic agent (Table 3-5).

Clinical Approach

The principles of diagnosis and treatment of opportunistic infection are basically similar to those used for other forms of infectious illness, but application of these principles is somewhat unique. The physician must be able to anticipate the onset of opportunistic infection and to recognize its presence even in the absence of classic signs and symptoms. While on occasion it may be necessary to institute antimicrobial therapy before having the advantage of an exact etiologic diagnosis, the frequent use of cultural and other diagnostic techniques must assume an importance far beyond their current scope.

In this situation a close reciprocal relationship must develop between the clinician at the bedside and the microbiologist in the laboratory. The physician must alert the microbiologist to the possibility of an opportunistic infection; in return, the microbiologist must regard the isolation by culture of "contaminants" or saprophytes, especially if recurring, with caution and suspicion. Together, such a medical team must attempt to determine the significance of the presence of these organisms. An approach to the diagnosis of opportunistic infection must be based upon: 1) an awareness of the circumstances in which it occurs, 2) acceptance of the concept that virtually any microorganisms can cause disease if the host is susceptible, and 3) familiarity with clinical characteristics of opportunistic infections.

The opportunists do not produce disease in a haphazard manner; therefore approaches to diagnosis need not and should not be haphazard. Rather, opportunistic infection should be anticipated as a distinct possibility in every patient with a known derangement of host resistance. These individuals fall into a relatively limited number of categories, as outlined in Tables 3-3 through 3-5; as a general rule, the greater the defect in resistance, the greater the likelihood of opportunistic infection. Anticipation of such an infection does not mean waiting for the patient to manifest obvious signs that infection has developed; by such time, delay in initiating therapy may have been catastrophic. By anticipation is meant a careful, periodic, microbiologic evaluation of pertinent material for aerobic and anaerobic culture in concert with careful clinical evaluation of the patient before infection has become clinically evident. For example, in the patient receiving antimetabolites for lymphoma via an indwelling intravenous catheter, periodic blood cultures should be drawn at predetermined intervals; furthermore, the intravenous site should be cultured in a similar manner, as should the distal end of the catheter each time it is changed. Cultures of sputum, urine, and stool should also be obtained so that the quantitative and qualitative characteristics of the patient's flora are known. Such knowledge can be of significant importance, for the first subtle clue of opportunistic infection may be the evolution of a new, predominating organism in the indigenous flora, the appearance of a new or unusual organism, or the repeated recovery of the same "contaminant," even if only in small numbers.

The discovery of an infectious process may be particularly difficult in patients with depressed host resistance. First, the usual clinical and laboratory signs of infection (fever, chills, leukocytosis) may be absent, especially in the elderly or debilitated patient; this may result from existing therapy or from inability of the patient to respond in a normal fashion. Second, the underlying disease may mimic infection; such events as the recurrent fever of lymphoma or the rejection of tissue transplants may be difficult to differentiate from signs of infection.

In anticipating opportunistic infection, one must look for signs which may seem totally unrelated to the presence of infection. A gross generalization is that any change in the clinical course of the patient should be regarded with suspicion. Experience suggests that certain occurrences should cause concern: sudden or insidious changes in mood, emotional affect, or appetite; bizarre behavior; somnolence; and hyperventilation are but a few. Physical manifestations include unexplained hypotension; thrombophlebitis —especially if recurrent, resistant to therapy, and in an unusual location; or bruising and hypesthesia around operative wounds.

Once opportunistic infection is suspected, every attempt must be made to document its presence and identify its cause. A wide variety of microbiologic techniques may be necessary, and it must be remembered that opportunistic infection frequently involves a synergistic combination of organisms requiring different methods for identification. The interpretation of cultural findings is often most perplexing, but certain factors are helpful in establishing clinical significance. The repeated demonstration of the same microorganisms by culture and smear is fundamental. Polymorphonuclear leukocytes on smears from disease sites, especially if these cells are phagocytizing suspected organisms, are particularly significant. The site from which opportunists are recovered may be helpful in this regard.

Although opportunistic infection occurs in a multiplicity of loci, certain organisms manifest a predilection for specific sites in relation to the underlying deficit in host defense mechanisms. For example, recovery of the fungus *Mucor* from the nasopharynx of the ketoacidotic diabetic takes on special significance, as does the presence of this fungus in the sputum of a leukemic patient. Similarly, recovery of nonhemolytic streptococci from blood or urine has far different significance from demonstration of the organism in the mouth and gingival crevices.

Appearance of an identical opportunist in cultures made from multiple sites is also helpful in diagnosis. The use of biopsy material for cultural and microscopic diagnosis should also be given strong consideration if opportunistic infection is suspected. If the unrelenting progress of infectious disease can be halted, the value of information obtained by biopsy would outweigh hazards of such a procedure. Repeated biopsy and even exploratory surgery may be necessary to arrive at a correct diagnosis. Demonstration of a rise in antibody titer to the organism in question may be helpful in smoldering infections, but is of doubtful value in rapidly progressive disease or in patients with impaired ability to sustain an immunologic response.

Once an etiologic diagnosis has been established, specific therapy should be instituted rapidly and vigorously. In a patient with basic underlying defects in resistance to the opportunists, delayed or inadequate treatment can be a tragic mistake. The decision to initiate treatment may be extremely difficult. On the one hand, a cultured opportunist may be a mere contaminant of no real importance; while on the other hand, early subtle hints of a change in the clinical status of a patient may provide the only opportunity to initiate successful therapy even though an etiologic diagnosis is not immediately available. In such a dilemma, sound clinical judgment and an awareness of the fundamentals of opportunistic infection must be combined to prevent undue delay in treatment.

In summary, pathogenicity may still be defined as the ability of an organism to cause disease; however, because of deficiencies that may arise in host resistance, the potential for pathogenicity must be extended to all microorganisms that constitute the indigenous or exogenous body flora. Acceptance of this concept by the physician and a willingness to pursue evidence to substantiate a diagnosis of opportunistic infection are now a necessary part of optimal care for many patients, especially those whose host resistance has been altered by underlying disease or its modern management.

SUGGESTED READING

1. ALEXANDER JW, MEAKINS JL: Natural defense mechanisms in clinical sepsis. J Surg Res 11:148–161, 1971

2. GEWÜRZ H: The immunologic role of complement, Immunobiology. Edited by RA Good, DW Fisher. Stamford, Conn, Sinauer Associates, 1971, pp 95–103

3. KLAINER AS, BEISEL WR: Opportunistic infection: a review. Am J Med Sci 258: 431–456, 1969

4. NISONOFF A: Molecules of immunity, Immunobiology. Edited by RA Good, DW Fisher. Stamford, Conn, Sinauer Associates, 1971, pp 65–74

5. WAKSMAN BH: Delayed hypersensitivity: immunologic and clinical aspects, Immunobiology. Editer by RA Good, DW Fisher. Stamford, Conn, Sinauer Associates, 1971, pp 28–34

6. WEINSTEIN L, KLAINER, AS: Septic shock—pathogenesis and treatment. N Engl J Med 264:950–953, 1966

4

Staphylococci

Staphylococci are ubiquitous and exist in the air and dust and on most fomites; they are part of the normal flora of humans and animals. Under certain circumstances they are capable of causing a wide spectrum of infections of varying severity.

Staphylococci are gram-positive, nonmotile, nonsporing microorganisms approximately 1 μ in diameter; they characteristically occur in grape-like clusters (Figs. 4-1 and 4-2), but single cocci, pairs, and chains are also seen. Staphylococci uncommonly are encapsulated but are covered with a carbohydrate surface slime, which, when viewed by scanning electron microscopy, may extend between cells to give the appearance of intercellular bridges (Figs. 4-3 and 4-4).

CLASSIFICATION   Staphylococci are characterized grossly by the color of colonies formed on solid media. Differentiation of two species, S. *aureus* and S. *epidermidis,* is outlined in Table 4-1. Staphylococci are also characterized by whether they are hemolytic and elaborate the enzyme, coagulase, which clots plasma; most strains of S. *aureus* pathogenic for man are hemolytic and produce this enzyme. It should be noted, however, that some hemolytic, coagulase-positive staphylococci do not produce pigment; it has therefore become standard practice to classify all coagulase-positive strains as S. *aureus.*

To only a limited extent staphylococci are grouped by antigenic polysaccharides and proteins. The main classification is based on **phage typing.**

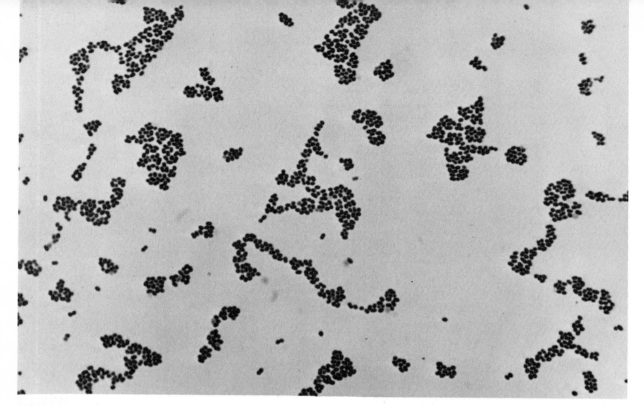

Fig. 4–1.
Staphylococcus aureus: gram stain of an 18-hour broth culture. (×900)

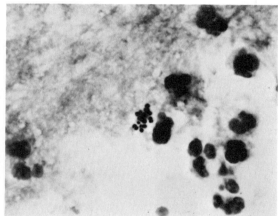

Fig. 4–2.
Staphylococcus aureus: gram stain of sputum from a patient with acute staphylococcal pneumonia. A cluster of staphylococci can be seen near pus cells. (×900)

Table 4-1. Gross Differentiation of Two Staphylococcal Species

Organism	Pigment	Coagulase reaction	Ferment mannitol	Hemolytic	Virulence
S. aureus	Yellow	Positive	Yes	Yes	Generally virulent
S. epidermidis	White	Negative	No	No	Generally non-virulent, but can cause disease under certain circumstances

Fig. 4–3.
Staphylococcus aureus: scanning electron microscopy reveals the typical spherical shape of the organism and grape-like clustering, as well as dividing cells (1), degenerating cells (2), and intercellular bridges (3), which are presumably due to the surface carbohydrate slime characteristic of many staphylococci. (Klainer AS, Betsch CJ: J Infect Dis 121:339–343, copyright [1970] The University of Chicago) (×10,000)

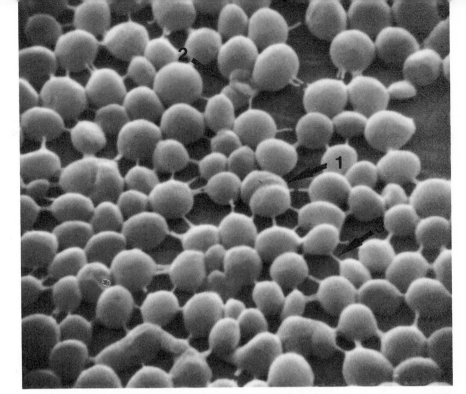

Fig. 4–4.
Staphylococcus aureus: scanning electron microscopy reveals intact (A) and ruptured (B) intercellular bridges of surface carbohydrate slime. (Klainer AS, Betsch CJ: J Infect Dis 121:339–343, Copyright [1970] The University of Chicago) (×20,000)

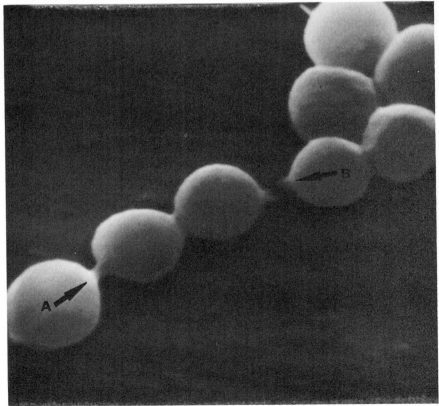

Bacteriophages are viruses which are bacterial parasites and are able to lyse their bacterial hosts. Phage type denotes the susceptibility of the organism to specific bacteriophages; it is a genetic characteristic based on surface receptors. Phage typing provides markers useful in epidemiologic studies, but it is applicable only to coagulase-positive staphylococci. The 80/81 phage type, for example, was implicated in the epidemic of hospital-acquired, penicillin-resistant staphylococcal infections encountered during the early 1960s.

CULTURAL CHARACTERISTICS

Staphylococci grow abundantly on all common media. Colonies appear creamy and yellow or white when grown aerobically at 37° C.

EXTRACELLULAR PRODUCTS

The precise factors which determine the virulence of staphylococci have yet to be identified; most likely virulence is based on a group of biologic characteristics that combine to make a specific strain virulent under certain circumstances. The only factor which correlates well with virulence in man is coagulase production.

Staphylococcci cause disease by eliciting an acute suppurative, necrotizing reaction characterized by abscess formation. In addition, staphylococci produce a variety of exotoxins and extracellular enzymes which are thought to be related to staphylococcal disease in man and animals, although the exact pathogenic mechanisms have not been elucidated.

Hemolysins. The most commonly elaborated toxins are the four immunologically distinct hemolysins—α, β, γ, and δ—which are species-specific. The most widely studied is the α-hemolysin, which is a potent hemolysin for rabbit erythrocytes (Fig. 4-5), causes a dermatonecrotic effect when injected into the skin of rabbits, is lethal when injected intravenously into rabbits and mice, and can injure rabbit and human leukocytes. The role of α-hemolysin in acute staphylococcal infections in man is unclear.

Leukocidin. Staphylococcal leukocidin is a nonhemolytic protein composed of two antigenically distinct, electrophoretically separable components: F (fast) and S (slow). Calcium ions are required for their action, which is related to leukocytic degranulation and results in death of or damage to the leukocytes.

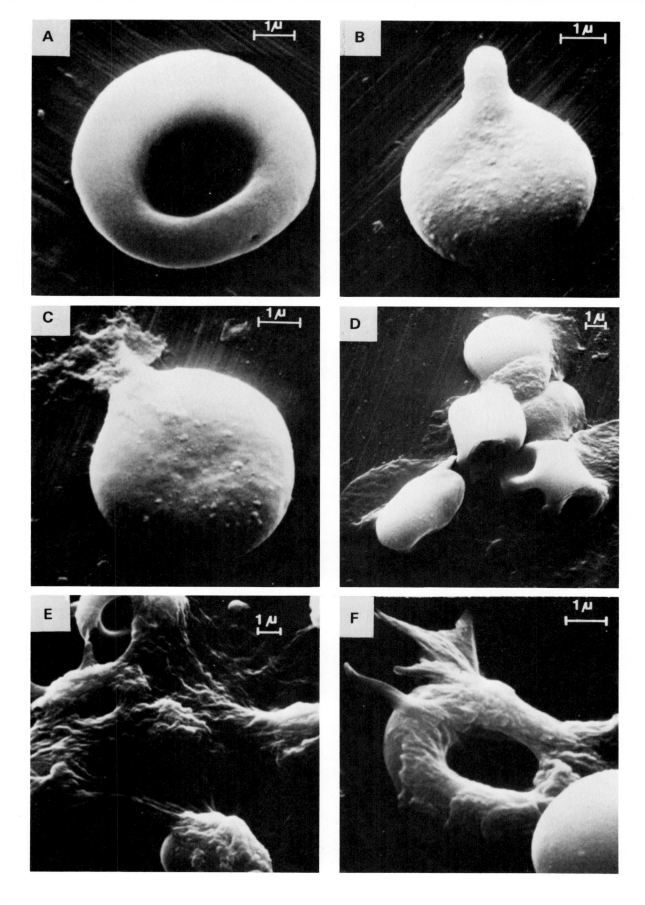

Enterotoxin. Some strains produce an enterotoxin which, when ingested, causes the syndrome of acute staphylococcal food poisoning.

Coagulase. Coagulase is an extracellular enzyme; staphylococci are the only bacteria that produce it. Coagulase causes citrated or oxalated plasma to coagulate and purified fibrinogen to clot in the presence of coagulase-reacting factor in plasma. Seven antigenically distinct coagulases have been identified.

Staphylokinase. Most coagulase-positive staphylococci produce a fibrinolytic enzyme, staphylokinase, which catalyzes the conversion of plasminogen to plasmin, a protease normally present in human plasma.

Hyaluronidase. Most pathogenic strains of staphylococci produce hyaluronidase, an extracellular enzyme which has a striking lytic effect on the ground substance of connective tissue and may play some role in the "spread" of staphylococcal infections. In general, staphylococci produce less hyaluronidase than do group A streptococci.

STAPHYLOCOCCAL DISEASES

S. aureus causes a wide spectrum of acute as well as several chronic infections in man.

Skin Infections

Staphylococcal furuncles and carbuncles represent localized skin infections which generally are not associated with systemic symptoms or gangrenous complications. Wound infections may be characterized by tissue necrosis, suppuration, and microabscess formation and may result in systemic spread via bacteremia.

Bacteremia

Staphylococcal bacteremia most commonly results from a portal of entry in the skin, although no obvious focus may be demonstrable. Staphylococcal bacteremia can be a rapidly fatal disease and is usually characterized by metastatic infection to many areas of the body including the meninges, endocardium, bones, joints, lungs, and kidneys.

Pneumonia

Staphylococcal pneumonia is never a primary infection in an otherwise healthy person, but most frequently is superimposed on a viral infection of the respiratory tract, especially influenza, or as a sequela of staphylococcal bacteremia. There are four types of staphylococcal pneumonia: 1) bronchopneumonia; 2) lobar pneumonia (occasionally accompanied by empyema); 3) interstitial pneumonia; and 4) diffuse bilateral bronchopneumonia (generally the result of bacteremia). Staphylococcal pneumonia is characterized by necrosis and microabscess formation; microabscesses coalesce, and consolidation results. Subpleural abscesses may rupture to cause empyema or pus in the pleural space. If a necrotizing lesion causes

rupture of air spaces, a pyopneumothorax results. Spread to the
num, the pericardium, and the blood may be seen in overwhelmir

Endocarditis

Staphylococcal bacteremia may result in acute necrotizing, ulcerating
lesions of the endocardium and rapid destruction of cardiac valves. It has
become a much feared catastrophic complication following cardiac surgery.

**Chronic Staphylococcal
Infection**

Although most staphylococcal infections are acute, several, such as
osteomyelitis, botryomycosis (chronic nodular subcutaneous staphylococcal
abscesses), chronic furunculosis, and perinephric abscess may be indolent
and chronic.

**Other Staphylococcal
Diseases**

Staphylococcal food poisoning is an intoxication, i.e., it is the result
of ingestion of preformed staphylococcal enterotoxin. It is characterized by
an incubation period of 4–24 hours (generally shorter than that of salmonella and shigella gastroenteritis), severe nausea, vomiting, abdominal
pain, diarrhea, and prostration.

Acute staphylococcal enterocolitis, on the other hand, is an infection of
the gastrointestinal tract characterized by invasion by the staphylococci
already inhabiting the patient's gut. It can lead to bacteremia and metastatic infection. Staphylococcal enterocolitis generally occurs in debilitated
patients following oral broad-spectrum antimicrobial agents. Diagnosis is
made by demonstrating the organism in gram stains of the stool; gram-
positive cocci are seen in large numbers almost to the exclusion of all other
stool flora.

Certain strains of phage group 2 have been associated with a spectrum of
dermatologic disease, the "staphylococcal scalded-skin syndrome" (e.g. Rit-
ter's syndrome or toxic epidermal necrolysis), now thought to be due to a
distinct staphylococcal toxin termed "exfoliatin" or "staphylococcal exfolia-
tive toxin."

**Infections Due To
*S. epidermidis***

S. epidermidis is a nearly constant inhabitant of the human skin; it is also
found frequently in the nose, throat, mouth, external auditory canal, conjunctivae, vagina, urethra, and feces of infants. Contamination of single
cultures by *S. epidermidis* is not uncommon; but when recovered repeatedly
from the same body fluid or diseased tissue, this organism must be considered the etiologic agent of disease. Septicemia due to *S. epidermidis*
almost always has recognizable predisposing factors. *S. epidermidis* has
been implicated in about 1% of cases of subacute bacterial endocarditis,
producing clinical illness similar to that caused by *Str. viridans*. It is one of
the organisms commonly implicated in endocarditis following cardiac
surgery. Urinary tract infections due to this organism are generally benign
and almost always can be related to antecedent manipulative procedures.
This organism has been estimated to produce about 4% of postoperative
wound infections, many of which clear spontaneously in 1 to 2 weeks

without antibiotic therapy. It should be emphasized that true infection with *S. epidermidis* usually is identified by multiple positive cultures, and that one should not be misled by the occasional contaminated culture.

ECOLOGY OF STAPHYLOCOCCAL INFECTIONS

Many persons carry staphylococci on the skin or in the nasopharynx. In some the carrier state may be transient; in others it is intermittent; and in a few, the organisms are found on an almost permanent basis. Continued exposure to environments in which staphylococci exist in high density, i.e., hospitals, or repeated exposure to broad-spectrum antimicrobial agents increase the chance of becoming a carrier.

Although a frightening increase in staphylococcal infections was observed during the early 1960s, this has become a problem of decreasing significance, in part because of the availability of an increasing number of potent and effective antistaphylococcal drugs. Still staphylococcal infection remains a serious threat in newborn nurseries, in the elderly with underlying debilitating diseases, in persons with immunologic deficiency diseases, and in those receiving x-radiation, antimetabolites, antimicrobial agents, and corticosteroids.

IMMUNITY TO STAPHYLOCOCCAL INFECTION

The role of the immune response in resistance to or recovery from staphylococcal infections is unclear. Normal adults possess antibodies to a variety of staphylococcal antigens and extracellular products, but this does not seem to prevent staphylococcal infection, and protective immunity does not appear to follow staphylococcal infection as it does a variety of other bacterial diseases.

SUGGESTED READING

1. CLUFF LE: Cellular reactions in the pathogenesis of staphylococcal infection. Ann NY Acad Sci 128:214–230, 1965
2. DUBOS R: Staphylococci and infection immunity. JAMA 184:1038–1039, 1963
3. FEKETY FR: The epidemiology and prevention of staphylococcal infection. Medicine (Baltimore) 43:593–613, 1964
4. KOENIG MG: Staphylococcal infections—treatment and control, Disease-a-Month. Chicago, Year Book Publishers, 1968, pp 1–36
5. NAHMIAS AJ, EICKHOFF TC: Staphylococcal infections in hospitals—recent developments in epidemiologic and laboratory investigation. N Engl J Med 265:74–81, 120–128, 177–182, 1961
6. RAMMELKAMP CH, MORTIMER EA, WOLINSKY E: Transmission of streptococcal and staphylococcal infections. Ann Intern Med 60:753–758, 1964
7. ROGERS DE: Staphylococcal infections, Disease-a-Month. Chicago, Year Book Publishers, 1958

Pneumococci

Pneumococci (*Diplococcus pneumoniae*) are pyogenic cocci which may be part of the normal flora of the upper respiratory tract of man. At certain times of the year, especially the winter months in colder climates, as many as 40% of the population may "carry" the organism in the nose and throat. Pneumococci are the commonest agent of bacterial pneumonia in man and can cause otitis media, sinusitis, and meningitis.

MORPHOLOGY   Pneumococci are encapsulated, nonmotile, nonsporing gram-positive diplococci which typically are lancet- or helmet-shaped and have a tendency to form short chains in sputum and pus (Figs. 5-1 through 5-3). Because aging, loss of viability, and exposure to appropriate antimicrobial agents may alter gram-staining characteristics, other criteria are also useful in differentiating the pyogenic cocci: Pneumococci possess short, parallel axes; neisseriae have long, parallel axes; and staphylococci and streptococci have axes of equal length due to their spherical shape when viewed by light microscopy (Fig. 5-4). Nevertheless, it is important to remember that morphologic characteristics, under the best of circumstances, provide only a crude and tentative means of identification which must be substantiated by culture.

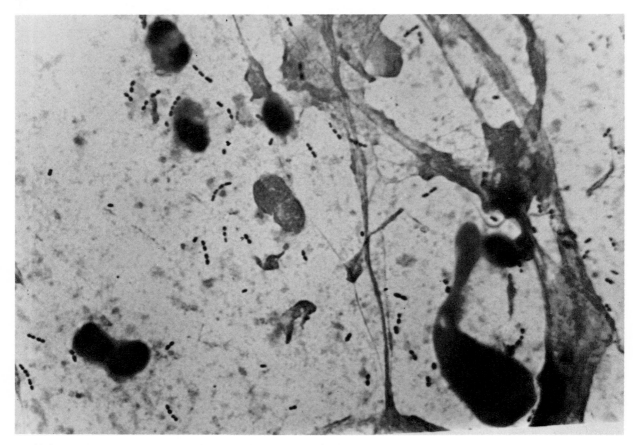

Fig. 5–1.
Gram stain of sputum from a patient with pneumococcal pneumonia. Polymorphonuclear leukocytes and a single predominating organism, pneumococci, are characteristic of pneumococcal pneumonia. Typical lancet- or helmet-shaped diplococci appearing as single pairs or in short chains are typical of pneumococci in sputum. (×1200)

Fig. 5–2.
Gram stain of spinal fluid from a patient with pneumococcal meningitis. Typical diplococci are seen around pus cells. (×900)

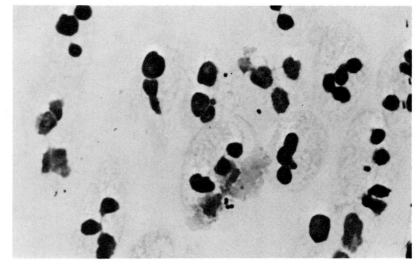

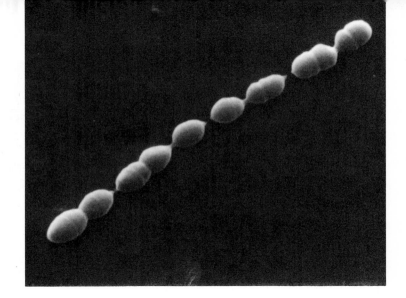

Fig. 5-3.
Scanning electron micrograph of type 3 *Diplococcus pneumoniae*. The organism is lancet- or helmet-shaped and typically occurs as diplococci in chains of varying length. (×10,000)

Fig. 5-4.
Axes of the pyogenic cocci. Pneumococci are characterized by short parallel axes; neisseriae by long parallel axes; staphylococci and streptococci by axes of equal length reflecting their spherical shape.

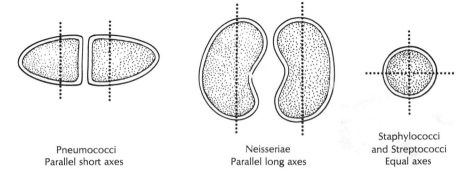

Pneumococci
Parallel short axes

Neisseriae
Parallel long axes

Staphylococci
and Streptococci
Equal axes

Fig. 5-5.
Scanning electron micrograph of the Quellung reaction. This type 3 pneumococcus has been exposed to type-specific anticapsular antibody, causing rounding and swelling of the organism. Compare with Figure 5-3. (×10,000)

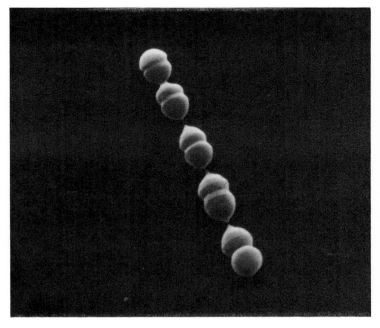

CULTURAL CHARACTERISTICS

Pneumococci are relatively fastidious, facultative anaerobes which produce a zone of α- or green hemolysis on blood agar and therefore must be differentiated from the α-hemolytic streptococci by the bile solubility and optochin sensitivity of the former; streptococci are not bile-soluble and are resistant to optochin. (Optochin is an alkaloid, ethylhydrocupreine hydrochloride, to which pneumococci are extremely sensitive.) Pneumococcal colonies are tiny, round, translucent colonies which are generally flat after 18 to 24 hours' incubation at 37°C and tend to become depressed or umbilicated because the center of the colony undergoes autolysis. This characteristic as well as the bile solubility test reflects the tendency of pneumococci to lyse spontaneously, especially in the presence of surface-active agents such as 10% bile or 2% sodium deoxycholate.

PNEUMOCOCCAL CAPSULES

Pneumococcal capsules are most easily demonstrated in India ink suspensions or by treatment with homologous type-specific antibody which combines with the capsular polysaccharide and causes it to become refractile (Fig. 5-5). This is called the **Quellung reaction.**

Pneumococcal capsules are composed of polysaccharides which are immunologically distinct for each of the many types identified. The capsule is related to pathogenicity via its antiphagocytic properties. Only smooth encapsulated strains are pathogenic for man and animals. Immunization with pneumococcal polysaccharide induces resistance to infection with the homologous type enhancing phagocytosis. In general, there is a rough correlation betweeen capsular size and virulence; those strains which produce the largest capsule, e.g., type 3, are most virulent for man and animals.

ANTIGENIC STRUCTURE

More than 80 serologic types (designated by Arabic numbers, i.e., types 3, 12, 14) of pneumococcci have been differentiated by their capsular polysaccharides. Other noncapsular (somatic) antigens include a poorly defined R-antigen and a carbohydrate C-substance, which are species-specific, and a type-specific M-protein (similar to type-specific M-antigens of group A streptococci, but antibodies to pneumococcal M-antigens are not protective). The C-substance is interesting in that it is precipitated by a β-globulin of serum in the presence of calcium ions and is the basis of the **C-reactive protein test,** a precipitation test to detect the presence of this protein in blood during the active phase of certain acute illnesses; it is widely used to follow the activity of a variety of inflammatory diseases such as rheumatic fever.

PNEUMOCOCCAL DISEASES

Pneumococci have been implicated as the etiologic agents of otitis media, sinusitis, epiglottitis, peritonitis (especially in persons with cirrhosis of the liver or the nephrotic syndrome), cholecystitis, suppurative arthritis, and osteomyelitis; but by far the commonest disease caused by these organisms is pneumococcal pneumonia, and the most severe is pneumococcal meningitis.

| Pneumococcal Pneumonia | Pneumococcal pneumonia accounts for 90–95% of all bacterial pneumonias. Although the death and complication rates have decreased since the advent of penicillin therapy, the incidence of pneumococcal pneumonia has not changed. It is more common during the winter months but occurs throughout the year. Pneumonia caused by the higher numbered types is more common, but the lower types, e.g., type 3, generally result in more virulent disease. As a rule, the disease is preceded by a nonspecific upper respiratory tract infection, but there may be no prodromal symptoms. Characteristically, the onset of the disease is sudden with shaking chills, fever, pleuritic chest pain, and cough productive of blood-streaked sputum, all occurring within a few hours; the onset, however, may be insidious. Pneumococcal pneumonia generally occurs as bronchopneumonia or lobar pneumonia, but the latter is less common since the availability of penicillin; the lower lobes are involved most frequently, but any part of one or both lungs may be affected. Pneumococcal bacteremia can be demonstrated in about one-third of patients. Abdominal pain is not uncommon, especially early in the course of the disease when the lung findings are minimal; this is more common with lower lobe pneumonia and is probably related to pneumonitis near the periphery of the diaphragm; the latter is innervated by the lower six intercostal nerves, which also innervate the upper abdomen. Complications (lung abscess, empyema, post pneumonic pleural effusion, atelectasis, bronchiectasis, bacteremia with subsequent endocarditis and meningitis) may be seen in the face of adequate antibiotic therapy but are more frequent when therapy has been inadequate or delayed. Most persons recover uneventfully with appropriate antibiotic therapy (penicillin), but 60–70% probably recover even in the absence of therapy. Certain factors, however, do predispose to greater mortality and morbidity: |

Age (neonates, the elderly)

More than one lobe involved

Pneumococcal infection elsewhere, e.g., sinusitis, meningitis

Bacteremia

Infection with more virulent lower types, especially type 3

Underlying diseases, especially congestive heart failure, renal failure, hepatic failure, immunologic deficiency diseases, blood dyscrasias

Alcoholism

Pregnancy

Leukopenia

Antimetabolite or corticosteroid therapy

Presence of complications

Inadequate, delayed, or improper therapy

| Pneumococcal Meningitis | Meningitis, the most severe of the pneumococcal infections, occurs in persons of all age groups. About half the cases are the result of pneumococcal bacteremia resulting from otitis media, sinusitis, purulent conjunctivitis, pneumonia, endocarditis, or cholecystitis; the other half appear as a primary meningitis, i.e., no obvious focus of infection can be demon- |

strated. In adults the most common meningitis associated with sinusitis, otitis media, and pneumonia is due to the pneumococcus. The cerebrospinal fluid is characterized by an increase in total white blood cells (mostly polymorphonuclear leukocytes), a moderate elevation of protein, decreased sugar (less than 50% of the simultaneous blood sugar level), and the presence of typical pneumococci; definite diagnosis, however, is dependent on demonstrating the organism in spinal fluid and/or blood by culture. The presence of large numbers of microorganisms with few polymorphonuclear leukocytes reflects a poor prognosis. The prognosis is best when pneumococcal meningitis is primary, and poorest when it is secondary to lobar pneumonia. Untreated pneumococcal meningitis is fatal; but even with penicillin therapy the mortality rate remains about 25% depending on the series of patients studied.

IMMUNITY TO PNEUMOCOCCAL INFECTION

Type-specific antibody can be demonstrated in the serum of patients with pneumococcal infection by the sixth or seventh day of the disease, and it generally remains for several months. Second attacks of pneumococcal infection are usually due to a new serologic type except where a persistent focus of infection exists (i.e., chronic sinusitis, bronchiectasis) or in patients with immunologic deficits.

Studies are now underway to develop pneumococcal vaccines, especially against the lower, more virulent types.

SUGGESTED READING

1. AUSTRIAN R, GOLD J: Pneumococcal bacteremia with especial reference to bacteremia pneumococcal pneumonia. Ann Intern Med 60:759–776, 1964

2. EPSTEIN M, CALIA RM, GABUZDA GJ: Pneumococcal peritonitis in patients with postnecrotic cirrhosis. N Engl J Med 278:69–73, 1968

3. HELDRICH JF JR: Diplococcus pneumoniae bacteremia. Am J Dis Child 119:12–17, 1970

4. JETER WS, MCKEE AP, MASON RJ: Inhibition of immune phagocytosis of Diplococcus pneumoniae by human neutrophiles with antibody against complement. J Immunol 86:386–391, 1961

5. MACLEOD CM: The pneumococci, Bacterial and Mycotic Infections of Man. Fourth edition. Edited by RJ Dubos, JG Hirsch. Philadelphia, Lippincott, 1965, pp 391–411

6. SHULMAN JA, PHILLIPS LA, PETERSDORF RG: Errors and hazards in the diagnosis and treatment of bacterial pneumonias. Ann Intern Med 62:41–58, 1965

7. WIFF RL, HAMBURGER M: The nature and treatment of pneumococcal pneumonia. Med Clin North Am 47:1257–1270, 1963

Streptococci

Streptococci are gram-positive cocci that occur characteristically in chains of varying length (Fig. 6-1). When viewed with the light microscope they appear as typical spherical cocci, but electron microscopy has shown them to be lancet-shaped and arranged in chains due to retention of cell wall material after cell division (Fig. 6-2); "tubular" forms are seen occasionally (Fig. 6-3).

Streptococci are widely distributed in nature; some are part of the normal flora of man and animals, whereas others cause disease either by direct infection or by eliciting an immunopathologic reaction in the host.

CLASSIFICATION Streptococci are classified by their hemolytic reaction, and by the presence of group-specific carbohydrates and type-specific proteins.

Hemolysis. Streptococci may be classified by grading the degree of hemolysis occurring around colonies on a blood agar plate (Table 6-1). Characterization of hemolysis is merely a crude method of classifying streptococci. The degree of hemolysis may vary depending on the strain of streptococcus, the type of blood used (sheep blood is best to demonstrate β-hemolysis), and whether colonies grow on the surface of or deep within the agar. In general, β-hemolytic streptococci are more invasive than those which manifest α- or γ-hemolysis.

Fig. 6–1.
Streptococcus pyogenes: typical chaining of streptococci is illustrated. The organisms are lancet-shaped. The diplococcic appearance is due to incomplete separation after cell division. The equatorial rings (1) reflect the site of new cell wall synthesis. There is a cell showing plasmolysis or shrinkage of the cytoplasm from the cell membrane (2). (Klainer AS, Perkins RL: JAMA 215:1655–1657, 1970) (×7500)

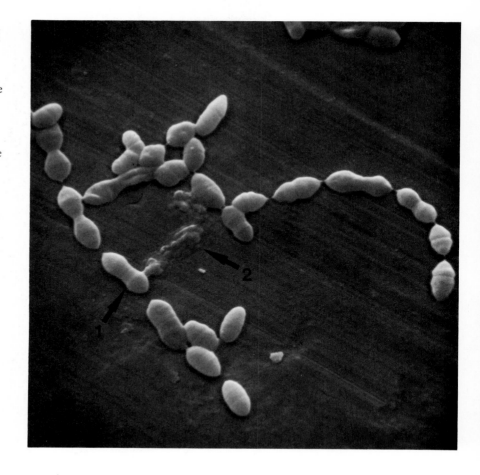

Table 6-1. Classification of Streptococci by Hemolysis on Blood Agar

Type of hemolysis	Appearance of zone of hemolysis	
	Gross	Microscopic
α	Green	Some intact red blood cells; green color due to presence of a reduction product of hemoglobin
β	Clear	No intact red blood cells present
γ	None	Red blood cells intact

Grouping. Streptococci are also classified by group-specific carbohydrate antigens in the cell wall. These C-carbohydrates are the basis for the Lancefield classification. Although many groups of streptococci may exist, 13 are of significance to man and animals. Groups are designated in capital letters (Table 6-2). There is no evidence that C-carbohydrates play a role in acute suppurative human disease; their role in the nonsuppurative complications of streptococcal infection, i.e., acute glomerulonephritis and acute rheumatic fever, is still questionable.

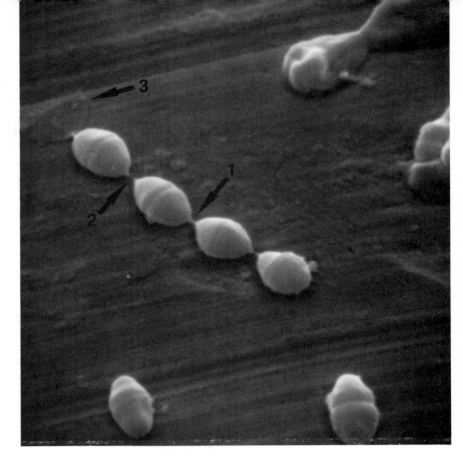

Fig. 6–2.
Streptococcus pyogenes: a typical chain of streptococci. Chaining is the result of retention of cell wall material between cells after cell division (1); separation of an intercellular bridge is also seen (2). At the upper end of the chain (3), part of a naked cell wall can be seen. (Klainer AS, Betsch CJ: J Infect Dis 121:339–343, Copyright [1970] The University of Chicago) (×15,000)

Fig. 6–3.
Streptococcus pyogenes, demonstrating a tubular form (arrow) that is simply dividing cells which have incompletely separated. (×10,000)

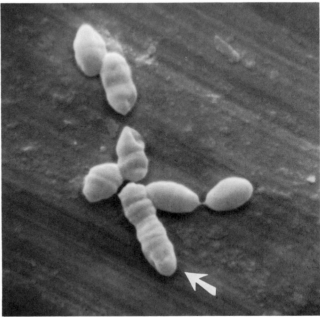

Table 6-2. *Classification of Streptococci by Group-Specific Carbohydrate (Lancefield Classification)*

Group	Significance to man and animals
A	Cause 95% of human streptococcal infections; most are β-hemolytic
B	Cause mastitis in cows, but some cases of bacteremia and meningitis have been reported in human neonates
C	Commonest group found in animals; can result in scarlet fever in man
D	Found in dairy products; have been seen as increasingly important pathogens in man, especially as a cause of urinary tract infections and endocarditis; may be β-hemolytic
E	Found in milk; a rare cause of pharyngitis in man
F	Have been isolated from the respiratory tract of man
G	Have been isolated from the upper respiratory tract of humans with scarlet fever and have been shown to be a cause of urinary tract infection in dogs; these organisms appear as very tiny colonies which are occasionally β-hemolytic
H,K	Have been found in the human upper respiratory tract
L,M	A cause of genital infections in dogs
N	Occur in dairy products
O	Occasional inhabitant of the respiratory tract of humans

Typing. Streptococci are typed by the nature of the type-specific M-proteins contained in their cell walls. Approximately 50 immunologic types have been described. Types are designated by numbers or proper names, and certain types are associated with an increased incidence of certain diseases (e.g., Red Lake strain and types 4 and 12 are nephritogenic strains—acute glomerulonephritis has been seen with increased frequency following infection with these types). Ordinarily five or six types are present in a community during interepidemic periods; the occurrence of a new predominant type generally heralds the onset of epidemic streptococcal infection. M-substance is a determinant of invasiveness: the more M-substance present, the more invasive is the organism. This relationship probably reflects the fact that M-protein is antiphagocytic. Antibody developed against M-substance is bactericidal (protective) and type-specific; this is in contrast to antibody against the group-specific capsular polysaccharide which is not protective.

The classification of streptococci can be summarized by using a typical organism as an example: group A (group-specific carbohydrate), type 12 (type-specific M-protein), β-hemolytic streptococcus (hemolytic reaction around the colony).

CULTURAL CHARACTERISTICS

Streptococci are more fastidious than staphylococci and grow best on blood agar. Streptococcal colonies are grayish, translucent, small (1–2 mm in diameter), nonpigmented colonies. Colonial morphology is similar for α-, β-, and γ-hemolytic streptococci. Streptococcal colonies appear similar to those of pneumococci but can be differentiated by the solubility of the latter in bile salts.

Many strains of hemolytic streptococci produce capsules. In group A streptococci the capsule is composed of hyaluronic acid. Capsules are demonstrable only in very young (2–4 hour) cultures.

On blood agar plates streptococcal colonies appear as one of three colonial types: 1) mucoid (glistening, moist colonies formed by strains which produce large capsules); 2) matt (rougher, dried colonies which are probably dried out mucoid colonies and do not reflect the presence of M-protein as previously thought); and 3) smooth (small, glossy colonies formed by nonencapsulated streptococci that usually produce large amounts of M-protein). In general, colonial morphology of group A streptococci is related to the hyaluronic acid capsule and not to M-protein.

EXTRACELLULAR PRODUCTS Group A streptococci produce a wide variety of extracellular products, many or all of which play a role in the pathogenesis of streptococcal diseases:

Streptolysin O. This is a hemolysin so designated because it is oxygen-labile (O) and is reversibly inactivated by atmospheric oxygen. Antibody to it (antistreptolysin O titer) is used as a retrospective aid in the diagnosis of recent streptococcal infection. Streptolysin O may be cardiotoxic.

Streptolysin S. This is a serum-soluble (S) hemolysin which is probably a poor antigen and therefore is not utilized as a diagnostic parameter of streptococcal infection.

Leukocidins. Leukocidins are labile factors, which in high concentration are toxic to white blood cells. These toxins, of which there are two, may be identical with the streptolysins.

Enterotoxin. Enterotoxin is an exotoxin which, if ingested, results in streptococcal food poisoning that may present with sore throat, nausea, vomiting, diarrhea, and a scarlet fever-like rash.

DPNase. This enzyme, diphosphopyridine nucleotidase (also NADase or nicotinamide adenine dinucleotidase), liberates nicotinamide from DPN. It may kill leukocytes that phagocytize strains of group A streptococci which elaborate this enzyme. Nephritogenic strains in particular produce DPNase, but there is no obvious relationship to the production of post-streptococcal glomerulonephritis. Anti-DPNase antibodies are found frequently in the sera of patients with recent streptococcal infection. DPNase may be cardiotoxic for animals and has been thought to play a role in the acute necrotizing myocarditis that occasionally develops after acute group A, β-hemolytic streptococcal pharyngitis.

DNAase. These enzymes depolymerize deoxyribonucleic acid (DNA). There are three immunologically distinct types (A, B, and C), which can be differentiated by electrophoresis. Although streptococcal DNAases are not cytotoxic because they cannot penetrate the cell membranes of living mammalian cells, depolymerization of DNA in pus may help to liquefy viscous purulent exudates. An enzyme preparation containing streptokinase and streptococcal DNAase (streptodornase) is commercially available for use as an enzymatic dibridement agent.

Streptokinase. This extracellular product of streptococci stimulates lysis of human blood clots by catalyzing the conversion of plasminogen to plasmin, a protease. Antistreptokinase antibodies are formed during infection with the group A streptococci.

Proteinase. Proteinase is an enzyme capable of destroying M-protein and other extracellular streptococcal proteins. It is active only at a pH of 5.5–6.5, and its role in the pathogenesis of streptococcal infections is unclear although it can cause necrotizing myocarditis in laboratory animals after intravenous administration.

Hyaluronidase. This enzyme lyses hyaluronic acid and therefore may alter the antiphagocytic properties of the streptococcal capsule. It was originally called "spreading factor" because of its ability to lyse the ground substance of connective tissue; whether this is of significance in the "spread" of streptococcal infection or in the pathogenesis of rheumatic fever is unclear. It is of interest, however, that human and streptococcal hyaluronic acids are chemically indistinguishable and that type 4 streptococcus, a strain which produces no hyaluronic acid, has not been associated with acute rheumatic fever.

Erythrogenic Toxin. Erythrogenic toxin causes the rash of scarlet fever. There are at least three antigenically distinct erythrogenic toxins—types A, B, and C—produced by different strains of streptococci. Erythrogenic toxins are produced by groups A, C, and G streptococci and some staphylococci. Although the exact mode of action of the erythrogenic toxins is not clear, they appear to act as capillary poisons, causing capillary dilatation (resulting in the striking erythema of the skin in scarlet fever), congestion in the capillary bed (resulting in punctate red spots in the skin), and increased capillary fragility (the cause of the petechiae and the bleeding lines in the skin observed in scarlet fever).

Dick Test

When erythrogenic toxin is injected into the skin of a susceptible person, it results in a localized area of erythema that is maximum at 24 hours (positive Dick test), indicating the absence of circulating antitoxin; in an immune person with circulating antitoxin, no erythema occurs (negative Dick test).

Schultz-Charlton Test

Intradermal injection of homologous antitoxin at the height of the scarlet fever rash causes local blanching. This has been used in confirming that an acute erythema is scarlet fever.

Disease due to infection with the streptococci is the result of one or a combination of events: 1) local injury at the site of invasion, 2) absorption of toxic materials elaborated by proliferating streptococci at the site of local injury, and 3) contiguous or systemic spread. Streptococci are usually transmitted from man to man by carriers, active cases, fomites, and via the air when the density of streptococci in the air reaches a critical level.

Pharyngitis

Group A, β-hemolytic streptococcal pharyngitis is the most common streptococcal disease and by far the most common of the bacterial pharyngitides. It is extremely difficult to diagnose streptococcal pharyngitis by clinical appearance alone. Typically it is characterized by sore throat, fever, leukocytosis, and localized tender lymphadenitis; the pharynx is magenta (purple-red) and frequently is spotted with purulent exudate; the presence of pinpoint petechiae at the junction of the soft and hard palate and on the uvula is a helpful diagnostic sign. The tonsils, if present, appear large and boggy and are also covered with exudate which wipes off easily. The diagnosis is tentatively made by the clinical appearance but must be substantiated by demonstrating the organism in cultures of material obtained by throat swab. There is no relationship, however, between the severity of the pharyngitis and the number of organisms isolated; in fact, no available cultural technique allows a 100% recovery rate of the organism.

The suppurative complications of streptococcal infection in the pharynx result from spread upward, downward, inward, or out onto the skin. Upward spread results in sinusitis, otitis media, mastoiditis, meningitis, or brain abscess; downward in laryngitis, tracheitis, and pneumonia; inward in bacteremia, with subsequent metastatic infection to any organ; and outward in paronychia, impetigo, cellulitis, and erysipelas.

Scarlet Fever

Scarlet fever is a disease state due to infection, usually acute pharyngitis, with an erythrogenic toxin-producing strain of streptococci in a susceptible host. The rash is punctate and typically starts behind the ears and spreads to the rest of the body; the face is usually spared except for the cheeks, and circumoral pallor is characteristic. The rash may be fleeting, or it may be very severe with petechiae and hemorrhagic cutaneous lesions. The tongue has the nonspecific appearance of a strawberry due to large, red papillae protruding through a whitish coating. Desquamation of the skin is typical as recovery progresses.

Cellulitis

Cellulitis is an infection of the subcutaneous tissues most commonly due to infection with the group A, β-hemolytic streptococci or staphylococci. It is characterized by localized pain, swelling, and redness which fades into the surrounding normal skin.

Erysipelas

In contrast to cellulitis, erysipelas is an infection of the dermis without involvement of the subcutaneous tissue but with acute lymphangitis. The lesion is red, warm, and painful, and is characterized by a slightly raised, serpiginous border which is sharply demarcated from the surrounding normal skin. Streptococci can be recovered occasionally from the lymphatic fluid in the advancing edge of the lesion. Eighty percent of erysipelas occurs on the face; it is usually bilateral and frequently involves the bridge of the nose and both cheeks. In some patients erysipelas can spread from the face upward over the forehead and scalp and downward over the neck, giving the patient a "swollen head." In children erysipelas of the abdominal wall can occur from infection of the umbilicus; genital infection can result from infection at or shortly after birth. Healing occurs from the center outward, and desquamation is common. Recurrence in the same or a different area is more frequent than with cellulitis.

Impetigo and Furunculosis

Impetigo is a primary superficial pyoderma characterized early by multiple discrete papulovesicular lesions on the skin which later become crusted. Impetigo often pursues a chronic course with individual lesions lasting a week or longer and cutaneous infection persisting for weeks or months.

Furunculosis is an infection of hair follicles; folliculitis and carbuncles are anatomic variants of furunculosis.

Non-suppurative Complications

The nonsuppurative complications of group A, β-hemolytic streptococcal infection are acute rheumatic fever and acute glomerulonephritis. Both are felt to be poststreptococcal immunopathologic reactions in the host. The exact mechanism whereby streptococcal infection leads to rheumatic fever has not been clearly elucidated; acute glomerulonephritis is thought to be mediated by soluble antigen-antibody complexes deposited on the basement membrane of the involved glomeruli.

SUGGESTED READING

1. DEIBEL RH: The group D streptococci. Bacteriol Rev 28:330–366, 1964
2. DENNY FW JR, PERRY WD, WANNAMAKER LW: Type-specific streptococcal antibody. J Clin Invest 36:1092–1100, 1957
3. DUMA RJ, WEINBERG AN, MEDREK TF, et al: Streptococcal infections: a bacteriologic and clinical study of streptococcal bacteremia. Medicine (Baltimore) 48:87–127, 1969
4. LANCEFIELD RC: Current knowledge of type-specific M antigens of group A streptococci J Immunol 89:307–313, 1962
5. MARKOWITZ AS, LANGE CF: Streptococcal related glomerulonephritis: I. Isolation, immunochemistry and comparative chemistry of soluble fractions from Type 12 nephritogenic streptococci and human glomeruli. J Immunol 92:565–575, 1964
6. RAMMELKAMP CH JR, MORTIMER EA JR, WOLINSKY E: Transmission of streptococcal and staphylococcal infections. Ann Intern Med 60:753–758, 1964
7. REINARZ JA, SANFORD JP: Human infections caused by non-group A or D streptococci. Medicine (Baltimore) 44:81–96, 1965
8. WANNAMAKER LW: The epidemiology of streptococcal infection. Streptococcal Infections. Edited by J McCarty. New York, Columbia University Press, 1954, pp 157–175
9. WANNAMAKER LW: Differences between streptococcal infections of the throat and of the skin. N Engl J Med 282:23–30, 78–84, 1970

Neisseriae

Although the two most important species of neisseriae are *Neisseria meningitidis* (the meningococcus) and N. *gonorrhoeae* (the gonococcus), several species are normal inhabitants of the upper respiratory tract and the distal few millimeters of the anterior urethra of humans. Man is the only natural reservoir of this organism.

Neisseriae are encapsulated, nonmotile, nonsporing, oxidase-positive, gram-negative cocci which are typically biscuit- or kidney-shaped and characteristically occur as diplococci with their long axes parallel (Fig. 7-1). The nonpathogenic neisseriae grow at 22°C and are generally non-fastidious; both the meningococcus and the gonococcus are more fastidious organisms, do not grow at 22°C, and are stimulated by an atmosphere of 5–10% carbon dioxide. The differential fermentation patterns are outlined in Table 7-1.

Two of the most important bacterial diseases of man, gonorrhea and meningococcal infections, are of sufficient significance to warrant thorough consideration.

MENINGOCOCCAL INFECTIONS

Serologically, meningococci are divided into five groups designated A, B, C, X, and Y according to group-specific capsular polysaccharide antigens (Table 7-2); the antigens can be demonstrated by agglutination or precipitin tests and by quellung reactions. In general, groups A, B, and C have

Table 7-1. Differential Fermentation Characteristics of the Neisseriae

Organism	Glucose	Maltose	Sucrose
N. catarrhalis	−	−	−
N. sicca	+	+	+
N. flavescens	−	−	−
N. meningitidis	+	+	−
N. gonorrhoeae	+	−	−

Table 7-2. Capsular Polysaccharide Antigens of the Meningococci

Group	Biochemical nature of the antigen
A	Mannosamine phosphate
B	N-Acetyl neuraminic acid
C	N-Acetyl neuraminic acid
X	Glucosamine-phosphate-glucose
Y	Glucosamine-phosphate, galactosamine

been associated with disease in man, whereas groups X and Y are considered nonvirulent. In this regard group-specific immunity should be acquired, but the exact status of immunity to the meningococci is not entirely clear. In the 1940s most meningococcal infections were due to group A organisms, in the 1950s to group B, and more recently to group C. In parallel, resistance to the sulfonamides has emerged so that at present approximately 60% of the organisms are resistant.

Meningococci cause disease via endotoxin, and there is some evidence that an exotoxin is also elaborated. The Shwartzman phenomenon can be produced with the meningococcus, but whether this reaction is related to clinical disease in man is uncertain.

Meningococcemia

The universal factor in all meningococcal infection is bacteremia. The portal of entry is usually the pharynx; the patient may or may not have a sore throat. Evidence is accumulating that the carrier state may induce protective antibody formation so that carriers, especially chronic carriers, are less likely to develop acute, overwhelming meningococcal infection. The conjunctivae are less frequent portals of entry, and meningococcal meningitis has been directly attributed to purulent conjunctivitis. Meningococcemia may be mild, severe with metastatic infection, fulminating and rapidly fatal, or chronic. The symptoms of meningococcemia characteristically include rash, fever, chills, myalgia, and arthralgia, the latter two being especially prominent. The rash is present in almost all patients who have meningococcemia; it starts typically as a pink, blanching morbilliform (measles-like) rash progressing to diffuse petechiae and purpura. Early in the course of the disease aspiration of the petechial rash allows demonstra-

Fig. 7–1.
Scanning electron micrograph of *Neisseria gonorrhoeae* demonstrating diplococcal arrangement with long axes parallel. (×10,000)

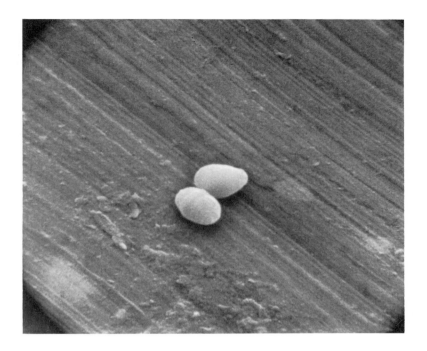

tion of the organism by smear and culture. In fulminating meningococcemia the purpuric areas become very large and progress to sedulations, large areas of hemorrhagic thrombosis with necrosis which may result in autoamputation of large areas of skin. Overwhelming meningococcemia usually results in death before metastatic spread can occur; in these cases death has been partly attributable to bilateral adrenal hemorrhage (Waterhouse-Friderichsen syndrome) and/or bleeding secondary to diffuse intravascular coagulation and depletion of clotting factors. Metastatic infection can involve any organ, but the meninges, joints, endocardium, pericardium, myocardium, and lungs are the most common sites. Chronic meningococcemia presents as repeated periodic episodes of fever, arthritis, and rash; it can terminate in meningitis.

Meningitis

Meningococcal meningitis is probably the most common of the bacterial meningitides. It has been called epidemic meningitis because it is the type of bacterial meningitis that can occur in epidemics; but most commonly there are just clusters of cases. Peak incidence is in persons less than 2 years of age and between 10 and 40 years. There is no obvious portal of entry, but the pharynx is the most likely focus. Bacteremia likely occurs in all cases but sometimes cannot be demonstrated; the presence of rash is helpful diagnostically, but it does not occur in all patients with meningococcal meningitis. Headache, fever, and signs of meningeal irritation are the most prominent symptoms. The cerebrospinal fluid findings are typical of any bacterial meningitis, i.e., elevated leukocyte count, low spinal fluid sugar/blood sugar ratio, and moderately elevated protein; it should be empha-

Fig. 7–2.
Gram stain of cerebrospinal fluid from a patient with meningococcal meningitis. Typical intracellular diplococci can be observed in the cytoplasm of some of the pus cells. (×900)

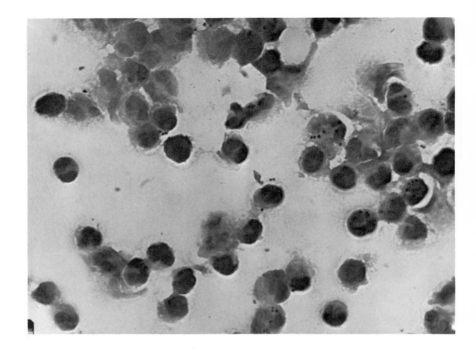

sized, however, that early in the course of the disease the cerebrospinal fluid findings may be normal. The diagnosis is made based on the clinical picture and gram stains of cerebrospinal fluid (Fig. 7-2) and petechiae; it is substantiated by demonstrating the organism in cultures of blood, spinal fluid, and petechial lesions.

Because of the developing resistance to sulfonamides and the tendency of acute meningococcal infections to occur in occasional epidemics and, more frequently, clusters, protective vaccines are being developed.

GONORRHEA

Gonorrhea is the third most frequently reported communicable disease in the United States. Yet the quarter million cases reported annually probably reflect only one-fifth to one-tenth the true number of cases that actually occur. Although the use of penicillin has been highly effective in the treatment of gonococcal infections, it has not resulted in an overall decrease in the incidence of gonorrhea.

Neisseria gonorrhoeae grows optimally under aerobic conditions at pH 7.2–7.6 at 35°–38°C. Most strains require an atmosphere containing 2–10% carbon dioxide to initiate growth. Primary cultivation of gonococci in the laboratory is difficult; not only do these organisms have fastidious growth requirements, but they are inhibited by a wide variety of substances present in common culture media. In addition, other bacteria frequently found in urethral and cervical secretions may grow more rapidly and obscure colonies of *N. gonorrhoeae*. A combination of growth-promoting and selective inhibitory substances for efficient recovery and identification of gonococci can be found in certain commercially available media, such as Thayer-Martin medium, which contains vancomycin, colymycin, and nystatin. Colonies of *N. gonorrhoeae* are translucent, raised, finely granular, mucoid, somewhat convex, and have lobate margins. They vary in size from pinpoint to 5 mm in diameter. The gonococcus is oxidase-positive, but many members of the genus *Neisseria* and other urethral and cervical bacteria also produce oxidase. The oxidase test is useful, however, when coupled with morphology, cultural characteristics, and sugar fermentation (Table 7-1). *N. gonorrhoeae* can be differentiated from other species of *Neisseria* found in the genital tract, i.e., *N. flava*, *N. catarrhalis*, *N. perflava*, and *N. sicca*, by differences in fermentation reactions and by the fact that these organisms, unlike the gonococcus, grow in the absence of blood, at 30°C, and appear as more hardy colonies.

Gonococcal Ophthalmia

Not all gonorrhea is contracted by the venereal route. The prepubertal child may become infected via articles contaminated with the genital discharge of an adult or other active source. The newborn may be threatened by gonorrheal ophthalmia, the most serious and historically the most common ocular infection during the neonatal period. Acute purulent gonorrheal conjunctivitis can progress, if untreated, to keratitis, with subsequent clouding of the cornea and blindness or to panophthalmitis with penetration and destruction of the globe. Gonorrheal ophthalmia generally occurs 3–7 days after birth. The disease is characterized by marked inflammation with edema and much purulent discharge. It must be differentiated from other causes of acute neonatal conjunctivitis, especially chemical conjunctivitis due to silver nitrate instillation and epidemic inclusion conjunctivitis. The latter generally occurs about 2 weeks after birth and is characterized by negative bacterial cultures and the presence of inclusion bodies in Giemsa-stained smears. A gram stain of the exudate in gonorrheal ophthalmia reveals characteristic gram-negative intracellular diplococci.

Vulvovaginitis

In general, gonorrheal infection is influenced by sex and by the menstrual status of the female. Prepubertal and postmenopausal women contract gonorrheal vulvovaginitis, an entity not seen in adult menstruating females. The lack of estrogen in the prepubertal and postmenopausal female allows the gonococcus to invade and infect the thin vulvovaginal membranes bathed in secretions of pH 6.8–7.4, which allows the microorganism to flourish. With the onset of menarche, estrogen causes the prepubertal membranes, which are only two to three cells deep, to thicken to a depth of 20 to 30 cells; these now become packed with glycogen, and the pH of the vaginal secretions falls to 3.5–4.5. The gonococcus cannot exist at a pH of less than 6.4. This explanation seems substantiated by the fact that newborns of mothers with gonorrhea do not get vulvovaginitis because of estrogen received from the mother, and by the fact that estrogen administration cures gonorrheal vulvovaginitis.

Genital Gonorrhea

Gonorrhea in the adult menstruating female often begins with acute urethritis manifested by dysuria, frequency, and purulent discharge. The disease may spread to Bartholin's and Skene's glands and result in abscess formation with swelling, redness, and pain. *Staphylococcus aureus*, streptococci, and other gram-negative organisms are more common causes of abscess formation in these glands than are gonococci, necessitating careful smear and culture of any purulent discharge obtained. Infection in the periurethral glands may become chronic and indolent. Cervicitis may occur alone or with urethral and periurethral infection. Cervicitis alone is more insidious in that the usual presenting symptoms of acute urethritis are absent and diagnosis is more difficult. From the cervix infection may spread to the tubes, resulting in salpingitis with abdominal pain and fever. The mucosa of the fallopian tubes becomes red, swollen, and covered by purulent exudate, which may escape into the peritoneal cavity to produce oophoritis, pelvic abscess, or acute peritonitis. Adhesions and scarring may occur and lead to pyosalpinx and sterility. In comparison, staphylococci and streptococci reach the tubes via the veins and lymphatics of the broad ligaments, resulting in thrombophlebitis, periphlebitis, lymphangitis, cellulitis, and even broad ligament abscess; although the walls of the fallopian tubes are thickened, the lumina remain patent, and sterility is much less frequent than with gonorrheal salpingitis. Acute pelvic inflammatory disease presents clinically with fever, chills, nausea, vomiting, lower abdominal pain, and tenderness in the adnexal regions. During the acute stage pelvic examination reveals either fixation of the uterus or pain on movement of the cervix. Chronic pelvic inflammatory disease with endometritis and salpingitis may be a sequel of the untreated or poorly treated acute process. This may be manifested by abdominal pain of varying

Fig. 7–3.
Gram stain of urethral discharge from a male with acute gonococcal urethritis. Clumps of typical intracellular diplococci can be seen in the pus cells in the center of the field. (×900)

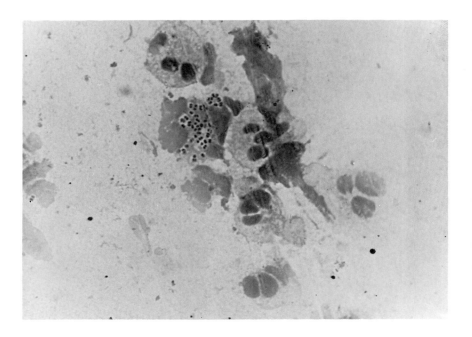

severity; it is often described as pressure or aching and worse before or during menstruation. The Curtis-Fitz-Hugh syndrome, or gonococcal perihepatitis, is seen only in the female. Organisms gain access to the peritoneal cavity via the fimbriated end of the fallopian tube and reach the liver via the gutter on the right side of the abdomen. A fibrinous exudate around the liver results in violin-string adhesions between the capsule of the liver and the undersurface of the diaphragm.

Especially important when considering gonorrhea in the adult menstruating female is the fact that the disease may be occult and asymptomatic. Gonococci are insidiously carried in the urogenital tract from which infection may be passed to a sexual partner.

In the adult male gonorrhea generally presents as acute urethritis 2–4 days after venereal contact. The entire length of the urethra, especially the anterior portion, is inflamed. There is dysuria and purulent urethral discharge; frequently on arising in the morning a drop of pus presents at the urethral meatus. A smear of the discharge reveals characteristic organisms in polymorphonuclear leukocytes (Fig. 7-3). If untreated, infection progresses posteriorly and may result in chronic posterior urethritis with stricture, prostatitis, seminal vesiculitis, and orchitis. The male, too, may acquire an asymptomatic infection and, in all likelihood, can transmit the disease in the absence of symptoms so long as sufficient viable organisms are present on contact.

Gonococcemia Gonococcal bacteremia is generally secondary to deep-seated infection and may mimic meningococcemia with fever, chills, and a petechial eruption. Acute bacteremia results in metastatic spread of infection. On the other hand, it may be chronic and mimic chronic meningococcemia with joint pain, morbilliform rash, and fever characterized by peaks every 48–72 hours. Bacteremia may result in an acute, necrotizing, ulcerative endocarditis. The gonococcus involves the right side of the heart, i.e., the tricuspid valve, more often than any other organism, but most frequently affects the aortic valve. Migratory mono- or polyarthritis involving primarily the larger joints may occur at any time during gonococcal illness. Tenosynovitis, especially of the wrists, dorsum of the hands and feet, areas of the internal and external malleoli, and insertions of the achilles tendons, is a frequent accompaniment of arthritis and is helpful in distinguishing gonococcal from other types of arthritis. Arthritis seen with gonococcal infection is of two types. Acute suppurative arthritis is seen in 3–5% of patients with gonococcal bacteremia and is manifested by purulent joint fluid containing organisms; it can result in the rapid and complete destruction of the joint. The second type of arthritis is more chronic, recurrent, and less destructive, and is probably due to a hypersensitivity reaction rather than metastatic infection; the joint fluid is usually sterile. There has, however, been a change in the incidence and clinical characteristics of gonococcal arthritis since the advent of antimicrobial therapy. Arthritis is now infrequently seen, and residual joint damage is uncommon in treated patients. In addition, recent observations suggest that gonorrhea with an acute septic course is associated with sterile arthritis because of early institution of therapy, whereas more indolent disease, characterized by a delay in seeking medical care, is associated with a higher incidence of culture-positive joint effusions. The association of arthritis with pericarditis further exemplifies the affinity of the gonococcus for serous surfaces. Acute purulent meningitis results from metastatic spread via the bloodstream. It is more frequent in males, but its true incidence is unknown because it is easily confused with the more common meningococcal meningitis from which it can be differentiated only by culture.

Skin Lesions
There are several skin manifestations of gonorrhea. The petechial and morbilliform rashes seen with bacteremia were mentioned above. A rare complication is keratosis blenorrhagica. A variety of skin eruptions are seen with chronic indolent gonococcemia; these typically appear during the first day of symptoms and may recur with each bout of fever. A hemorrhagic and vesiculopustular eruption which is tender in the early stages of development has been described. The fluid within these lesions is serous but may contain organisms. This type of lesion is most likely the result of bacterial embolization with subsequent septic infarction.

Carrier State
A less dramatic but equally important aspect of gonococcal infection is the carrier state. The carrier has active gonococcal infection and is capable of transmitting the disease in the absence of symptoms of acute or chronic gonorrhea. As gonorrhea has become more difficult to treat, the incidence of the carrier state has increased. It is seen predominantly in women, but is becoming more common in men and precludes using the disappearance of symptoms as adequate evidence for successful antimicrobial therapy.

Diagnosis
Diagnosis of gonorrhea depends upon the bacteriologic demonstration and identification of *N. gonorrhoeae*. In the male a gram stain of urethral discharge or prostatic secretions after gentle massage is helpful but not diagnostic (Fig. 7-3). Only 70–95% of positive smears can be substantiated by culture. In addition, members of the genus *Mima* or other neisseriae may be mistaken for *N. gonorrhoeae*. The fluorescent antibody technique has made rapid diagnosis more reliable.

In the female, smears are much less helpful because female patients with gonorrhea often have a negative smear. The most reliable method for diagnosis is to obtain multiple specimens for smear and culture from the vagina, urethra, cervix, and anal canal.

There is little doubt that there has been an increasing incidence of failure in the treatment of gonorrhea with penicillin. Most important is the changing sensitivity of the gonococcus to that antibiotic. Until recently the majority of gonococci were sensitive to 0.001–0.050 units/ml. of penicillin. At present, some strains are sensitive only to levels as high as 4.0 units/ml. In spite of this, penicillin still remains the treatment of choice.

Prevention   The basis of prevention is the identification and therapy of contacts of a known case of gonorrhea. Male patients especially should be questioned about their contacts because frequently their female sex partners are asymptomatic. Contacts of the past 3 weeks are significant. The use of condoms and good urogenital hygiene is also helpful. Prophylaxis against gonorrheal ophthalmia neonatorum is mandatory; the treatment of mothers cannot be relied upon as an adequate measure because infection of the newborn can result from asymptomatic mothers. Silver nitrate (1%) instillation or the use of some other ophthalmic antigonococcal agent at birth remains the *sine qua non* for prevention of this potentially blinding ocular infection.

Every patient with gonorrhea should have at least two serologic tests for syphilis the last 3 months after the patient's last known exposure. The effect of penicillin therapy and prophylaxis of gonorrhea on the ability to diagnose concurrent syphilis remains an enigma.

NONPATHOGENIC NEISSERIAE   Indigenous neisseriae (including the anaerobic gram-negative cocci classified as veillonellae) are found in the nasal and oral cavities, saliva, pharynx, anterior urethra, vagina, and lower intestinal tract. Although the many subspecies of indigenous neisseriae are usually harmless saprophytes, they may cause serious disease including endocarditis and meningitis. In the latter the spinal fluid rarely may appear green-yellow when meningitis is caused by pigment-producing neisseriae. Although most cases of meningitis occur without obvious underlying disease, a congenital defect may provide the portal of entry. Because many species of *Neisseria* are common inhabitants of the upper airway, it is especially difficult to differentiate between their role as members of the normal flora and that as the primary organism causing disease.

SUGGESTED READING

1. EICKHOFF TC, FINLAND M: Changing susceptibility of meningococci to antimicrobial agents. N Engl J Med 272:395–398, 1965

2. FELDMAN HA: Sulfonamide-resistant meningococci. Annu Rev Med 18:495–506, 1967

3. FELDMAN HA: Recent developments in the therapy and control of meningococcal infections, Disease-A-Month. Chicago, Year Book Publishers, 1966

4. MARTIN JE JR, LESTER A, PRICE EV, SCHMALE JD: Comparative study of gonococcal susceptibility in the United States, 1955–1969. J Infect Dis 122:459–461, 1970

5. SCHROETER AL, PAZIN GJ: Gonorrhea. Ann Intern Med 72:553–559, 1970

6. WOLFE RE, BIRBARA CA: Meningococcal infections at any army training center. Am J Med 44:243–254, 1968

Corynebacteria

Corynebacteria are gram-positive, nonmotile, nonspore-forming, unencapsulated aerobic rods; they often are club-shaped (Fig. 8-1) and possess irregularly staining granules (metachromatic granules, Babes-Ernst bodies). In smears they are often seen in typical palisade ("picket fence") or cuneiform ("Chinese letter") arrangements, i.e., they line up in parallel rows or form sharp angles to one another. Several species are part of the normal flora of the human skin and mucous membranes (these are generally called diphtheroids), whereas one species, *Corynebacterium diphtheriae* (the diphtheria bacillus), produces one of the most powerful exotoxins known and causes diphtheria in man. The only known reservoir of *C. diphtheriae* in nature is man.

CULTURAL CHARACTERISTICS

Corynebacteria appear as small granular gray colonies on Löffler's coagulated serum medium. On tellurite agar the colonies are dark gray or black because of the reduction of the tellurite to tellurium. Three morphologically distinct types of *C. diphtheriae* occur on this medium: var. *gravis*, var. *mitis*, and var. *intermedius*; their characteristics are outlined in Table 8-1. Corynebacteria also grow on most ordinary laboratory media. Acid, but not gas, is formed from the carbohydrates fermented (Table 8-1). There is no absolute correlation between the severity of the disease and the strain involved.

Fig. 8–1.
Scanning electron micrograph of *Corynebacterium diphtheriae* demonstrating typical clubshaped rod. (×10,000)

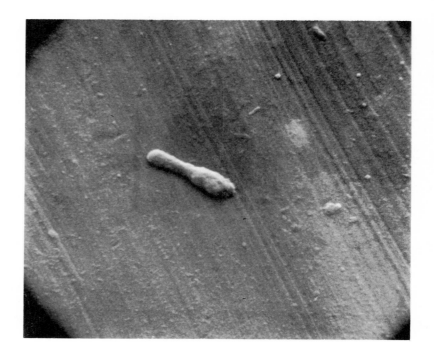

DIPHTHERIA TOXIN Only those strains of *C. diphtheriae* that are lysogenic (contain a low concentration of bacteriophage) for prophage-β or a closely related bacteriophage produce diphtheria toxin; if a toxigenic strain loses its phage, it becomes nontoxigenic. In addition, toxin production is dependent upon an optimum concentration of iron (either ferrous or ferric) in the environment; whereas the presence of iron is necessary for multiplication, toxin production occurs only when environmental and intracellular iron concentrations are at very low levels. The toxins produced by all strains of *C. diphtheriae* are immunologically identical, a factor which has been of great importance in controlling the disease. The exact pathogenetic mechanism of diphtheria toxin in man has not been entirely elucidated, but it is known to cause necrosis and hemorrhage in the adrenal glands, heart, liver, and kidneys when injected into susceptible animals. At the subcellular level diphtheria toxin interferes with protein synthesis at least in one way by preventing the incorporation of amino acids into protein by inhibiting the transfer of amino acids from soluble RNA to the growing peptide chain; this is a nicotinamide adenine dinucleotide (NAD)—dependent reaction. The toxin also interferes with the rate of oxidation of long-chain fatty acids.

DIPHTHERIA Most of the clinical picture of diphtheria is due to the effects of the toxin. The organism is acquired from a carrier or a person with the active disease. After an incubation period of 2–5 days, symptoms begin. Symptoms occur based on the extent of the local growth of the organism and its production of toxin, with its local and distant effects.

Table 8-1. Characteristics of Corynebacteria Diphtheriae

Organism	Cell morphology	Appearance on tellurite agar	Appearance in broth	Hemolysis	Fermentation			Effect on tissue
					Glucose	Sucrose	Starch	
C. diphtheriae var. *gravis*	Short rods	Gray, "daisy head" colonies	Form a pellicle	−	+	−	+	Necrosis, hemorrhage
C. diphtheriae var. *mitis*	Long rods, occ. granule at each end	Small, shiny, black colonies	Grow diffusely	+	+	−	−	Little
C. diphtheriae var. *intermedius*	Long, clubbed rods with cross barring	Medium-sized, black, dull colonies	Settle as granular sediment	−	−	−	−	More than mitis variety; less than gravis variety

Faucial Diphtheria   Diphtheria in the throat and tonsils first appears as a discrete whitish exudate in the crypts of the tonsils; at the start of the disease the exudate wipes off easily without bleeding. As the exudate spreads, a thin membrane forms which becomes thick, hard, and adherent, and wipes off only with difficulty and resultant bleeding. The organism can be demonstrated in smears of the exudate and membrane. Every case of membranous pharyngitis should be suspected to be diphtheria until smears and cultures prove otherwise. In general, severe sore throat and high fever are not characteristic of diphtheria; this is helpful in differentiating it from streptococcal pharyngitis or infectious mononucleosis. The course of faucial diphtheria is outlined in Figure 8-2. Extension may result in respiratory tract obstruction and death. Bloodstream invasion also may occur. Complications are due to toxin production and toxemia as well as extension. Toxic myocarditis occurs in about 65% of cases; infections caused by both the mitis and gravis varieties of the organism cause the same incidence of myocarditis, but death occurs more frequently with the gravis variety. Recovery from diphtheritic myocarditis occurs via fibrosis; persons who recover do not have entirely normal hearts. The peripheral nervous system may be involved in three ways: 1) peripheral neuritis of the cranial nerves early in course of the disease; 2) peripheral neuritis during the second and third weeks of the disease, with motor but not sensory involvement; and 3) an infectious polyneuritis-like picture occurring 2–3 months after the onset of symptoms. Encephalitis, kidney necrosis, and thrombocytopenia are other possible complications.

Nasal Diphtheria   Nasal diphtheria may be chronic, lasting for months. The membrane occurs in the nares and nose. Toxin is generally not absorbed.

Laryngeal Diphtheria   The laryngeal form of diphtheria may present as a croup-like illness. The membrane may completely obstruct the respiratory tract and result in death.

Figure 8-2. The Course of
Faucial Diphtheria

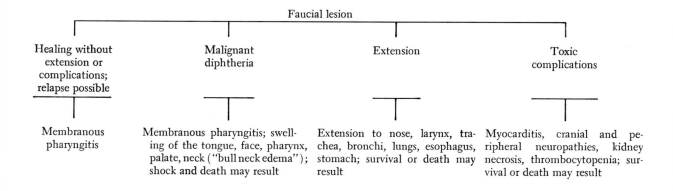

Figure 8-2. The Course of Faucial Diphtheria

Skin Diphtheria Diphtheria of the skin is a chronic, indolent form of the disease, generally presenting as shaggy ulcerations covered with a brown or grayish membrane. It is more common in tropical climates and can be a source of faucial diphtheria. If caused by toxin-producing strains, myocarditis and peripheral neuritis may result.

Other Types of Diphtheria The genitalia and the conjunctivae may also be sites of diphtheria.

IMMUNITY Resistance to diphtheria is largely dependent on the presence of specific neutralizing antitoxin in the blood and tissues. Diphtheria generally occurs in persons without or with very low levels of antitoxin. The most severe disease usually occurs in persons with blood antitoxin levels less than 0.01 units/ml; if the blood level is greater than 0.1 units/ml, death is uncommon. Immunity to diphtheria may be active (in response to immunization or the natural disease, which is usually followed by lasting immunity) or passive (via the administration of preformed specific antitoxin, which is part of the treatment for the disease along with penicillin or other appropriate antibiotics to eliminate the organisms producing the toxin).

Schick Test The Schick test is based upon the injection of 1/50 minimum lethal dose for guinea pigs into the skin of one forearm of the human subject and an identical amount of heated toxin into the other arm as a control. The results and interpretation of the Schick test are outlined in Table 8-2.

IMMUNIZATION Primary immunization is usually performed during the first year of life with fluid toxoid (a filtrate of a broth culture of a toxigenic strain treated with 0.3% formalin until toxicity is absent). Boosters are administered at

Table 8-2. Schick Test

Reaction	Morphology*	Interpretation
Positive	Toxin produces redness and swelling, which appears in about 24 to 48 hrs, increases for several days and then fades slowly; control site no reaction	Susceptibility to diphtheria toxin; inadequate circulating antitoxin
Negative	No reaction with toxin or control	Adequate amount of circulating antitoxin
Pseudoreaction	Redness and swelling with both toxin and control; reaches maximum in 48 to 72 hrs and then fades	Hypersensitivity reaction to toxin indicating immunity, usually high level, plus hypersensitivity
Combined	Redness and swelling with both toxin and control, but former reaction continues after that of the control subsides	Hypersensitivity to toxin and other proteins; antitoxin is either absent or present in low concentration

* The test is read at 24 and 48 hours and again in 6 days.

ages 1 year, 3–4 years, and 6–8 years, and then intermittently throughout life. Alum-precipitated toxoid (toxoid prepared as above but precipitated with 1–2% potassium alum) can also be used, but this results in hypersensitivity reactions more frequently than when fluid toxoid is used. Diphtheria toxoid is commonly combined with tetanus toxoid and pertussis vaccine in a single injection.

Moloney Test

Reimmunization, especially of older children and adults, may cause serious hypersensitivity reactions. Intradermal injection of 0.1 ml of a 1:10 dilution of the toxoid (Moloney test) is helpful in evaluating the likelihood of such a reaction. The development of a local reaction suggests that the toxoid should be administered cautiously.

DIPHTHEROIDS

Certain corynebacteria, such as C. *pseudodiphtheriticum* and C. *xerose*, are called diphtheroids and are normally found on the mucous membranes of the respiratory tract, conjunctivae, and vagina. While these organisms often contaminate other cultures, they may also cause disease. Cases of brain abscess and endocarditis have been reported. Endocarditis due to diphtheroids has been described after cardiopulmonary bypass surgery for valvular heart disease. Diphtheroid endocarditis has also occurred following antibiotic therapy for subacute bacterial endocarditis of other etiology. The diphtheroids typify the clinical problem of opportunistic infection, since they are frequent contaminants of material obtained for culture. An awareness that these organisms can cause infectious disease and the ability to recover the organism repeatedly from the site of disease are the bases for diagnosis.

SUGGESTED READING

1. WEINSTEIN LW: The Practice of Infectious Diseases. New York, Landsberger Medical Books, 1958, pp 117–125

2. COLLIER RJ, PAPPENHEIMER AM JR: Studies on the mode of action of diphtheria toxin. J Exp Med 120:1007–1018, 1019–1039, 1964

3. KAPLAN K, WEINSTEIN LW: Diphtheroid infections of man. Ann Intern Med 70:919–929, 1969

Clostridia

The clostridia are gram-positive anaerobic spore-forming bacilli (Figs. 9-1 and 9-2). Most species are motile and demonstrate hemolysis on blood agar. The clostridia are natural inhabitants of the soil and the intestinal tracts of man and animals; but under the proper conditions they can be dangerous pathogens, being the causative agents of tetanus, gas gangrene, and botulism.

TETANUS   Tetanus is produced by *Clostridium tetani*. The organism is a slender rod which, when sporulation occurs, develops a terminal spore giving it its characteristic "drumstick" or "tennis racquet" appearance (Fig. 9-3). Destruction of tissue, typical of clostridial gangrene, is not a prime feature; all of the clinical manifestations of the disease are produced by a soluble exotoxin, tetanospasmin, which is elaborated by the vegetative form of *Cl. tetani* as it multiplies in injured tissues. Tetanospasmin is a protein with a molecular weight of about 67,000 and, next to botulinus toxin, is the most powerful bacterial poison known. *Cl. tetani* also produces a hemolysin, tetanolysin, but this substance does not contribute to the clinical picture of tetanus.

Cl. tetani is usually introduced into an area of injury in its spore form, since this is the form of the organism present in soil and intestinal contents. Disease does not develop unless the spore vegetates into the toxin-produc-

Fig. 9–1.
Clostridium species. Gram stain shows typical darkly stained rods. Within some of the lighter stained rods, empty spaces typical of spores can be seen. (×1000)

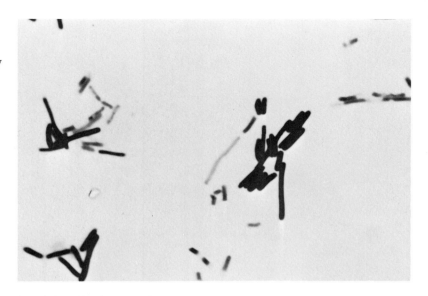

Fig. 9–2.
Scanning electron micrograph of a species of *Clostridium*. The flattened ends are due to washing prior to fixation of the preparation and are not part of the characteristic morphology. (×10,000)

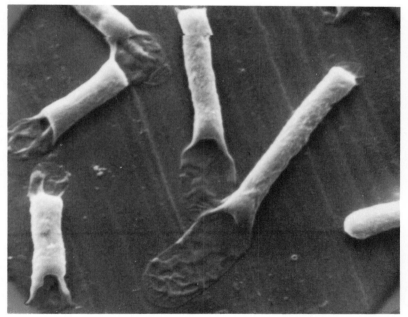

ing form of the organism. Tissue injury as well as an optimum oxidation-reduction potential and reduced oxygen tension locally are necessary for vegetation to occur; this is potentiated by tissue necrosis, the presence of foreign bodies, and suppuration in the area where the spores are introduced. The exact mechanism whereby tetanus toxin formed at the site of *Cl. tetani* growth is transmitted to the central nervous system is not entirely clear. Most of the available evidence suggests that the toxin is transported along elements of the peripheral nerves.

Fig. 9–3.
Clostridium tetani, illustrating the typical drumstick appearance due to a terminal spore. (×10,000)

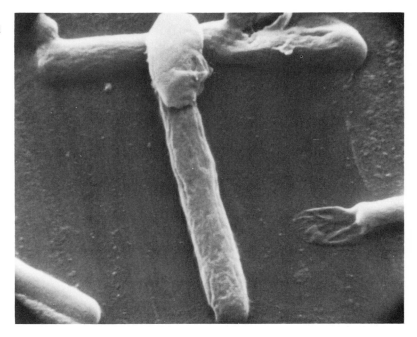

The pathophysiology of tetanus is also not well understood. In generalized tetanus the primary effect of the toxin is on the spinal cord, whereas in localized tetanus it is on the motor nerve endings, the peripheral nerves, or muscle fibers. In general, however, the complex polysynaptic reflexes involving interneurones are primarily involved; the major action of the toxin is probably to suppress the inhibitory action of the interneuronal system, resulting in a state of generalized hyperexcitability. The clinical features of tetanus are all related to the sustained contraction of muscle groups. Isolated groups of muscles or all of the major muscle groups may be excited.

The incubation period in humans is usually 3–21 days; however, it may be as short as 1 day or as long as several months. There appears to be a relationship between the site of injury and the interval before the onset of the disease; the longer the toxin must travel along peripheral nerves to reach the central nervous system, the longer the incubation period.

There are two forms of tetanus: generalized and local. Local tetanus is an uncommon form of the disease in civilians and may be easily overlooked. Its characteristic manifestation is a persistent and unyielding rigidity of the group of muscles in close proximity to the site of injury. It is frequently seen when antitoxin has been administered in a dose sufficient to neutralize circulating toxin but insufficient to prevent or inactivate significant local accumulation. Symptoms may persist for several weeks or even for a few months, finally disappearing without neurologic residual. Local tetanus may precede the development of generalized tetanus and is usually a mild disease with a low mortality rate (less than 1%).

Generalized tetanus is the most common form of the disease. In 80% of cases the portal of entry is an insignificant wound contaminated by tetanus spores which may then vegetate when the local tissue environment is favorable. Umbilical infection of the newborn is the lesion most commonly associated with tetanus neonatorum, a particularly lethal form of the disease. Injury to the scalp, face, eyes, ears, neck, and other structures of or near the head may predispose to the development of cephalic tetanus, a very virulent form of the disease.

Trismus is the presenting symptom in over 50% of cases of tetanus; restlessness, irritability, stiffness of the neck, or difficulty in swallowing are other common presenting symptoms. As the disease progresses, involvement of other mucle groups results in tonic contractions of the muscles of the jaws, face, neck, back and abdomen. Persistent trismus produces a characteristic facial expression, the so-called sardonic smile (risus sardonicus). The abdominal and lumbar muscles may become rigid as may those of the chest. Intense persistent spasm of back muscles may result in opisthotonus, which usually is associated with generalized seizures (tonic tetanospasms) unique to tetanus; there is a sudden burst of tonic contractions of muscle groups causing opisthotonus, flexion and adduction of the arms, clenching of the fists on the thorax, and extension of the lower extremities. Unfortunately, the patient is completely conscious during these episodes and experiences intense pain. Difficulty in swallowing leads to hydrophobia. Such seizure activity can be triggered by the slightest external stimuli, even a breeze or simply touching the patient. Glottal or laryngeal spasm may cause asphyxia.

Laboratory studies are of little value in the diagnosis of tetanus. Gram stains of the wound may reveal characteristic organisms. Culture of exudate or necrotic tissue, if present, in thioglycollate broth or chopped meat medium may reveal typical sporulated forms. The diagnosis of tetanus is based on a history of injury followed by the development of any of the syndromes described above.

Treatment of tetanus includes: 1) neutralization of circulating tetanus toxin before it reaches the nervous system by administering specific antitoxin (human antitoxin is now available and has eliminated the potential development of serum sickness, a risk inherent in the use of horse serum); 2) eradication of the toxin-producing Cl. tetani from foci of infection by the use of appropriate antibiotics (in most cases, penicillin) and surgical debridement; and 3) intensive supportive care of the patient in a quiet environment with the adequate use of sedation, vigorous treatment of seizure activity, and maintenance of an adequate airway.

Most important, however, is that tetanus is a preventable disease. Active immunization is readily achieved by means of either alum-precipitated or fluid toxoid—usually given during childhood in combination as DPT (diphtheria, pertussis, tetanus). Tetanus boosters should be given approximately every 5 years. In certain circumstances when the immune status of an individual is uncertain after deep puncture wounds and grossly contaminated wounds, immediate protection may be necessary and accomplished by a booster dose of toxoid and the administration of specific antitoxin.

Unlike tetanus, which is produced by a single toxin elaborated by the single bacterium *Cl. tetani*, most clostridial infections involve several species elaborating a variety of substances. Many species of clostridia may be involved, but the most common are *Cl. perfringens*, *Cl. novyi* and *Cl. septicum*. *Cl. perfringens* is the most important species associated with gas gangrene and has been the most widely studied. It produces several toxins, the basis for division of the species into six types. Only type A is of particular importance in human disease.

Gas gangrene results from clostridial infection, first in damaged muscle and later in healthy muscle. Injured muscle rendered anoxic by damage to the nutrient blood supply provides an ideal anaerobic environment for the growth of clostridia, but other factors, including a favorable oxidation-reduction potential and optimum calcium ion concentration, are necessary for adequate toxin production to occur, the result being gas gangrene. The invasion of muscle and the toxemia of gas gangrene is basically the result of one or more clostridial toxins. The toxins of *Cl. perfringens* are outlined in Table 9-1. α-Toxin is the most important, but it is likely that a combination of specific actions of individual toxins are involved in the pathogenesis of gas gangrene. True gas gangrene is clostridial myonecrosis and myositis, which should be distinguished from simple contamination by clostridia, from clostridial cellulitis, or from other anaerobic or synergistic infections of skin, subcutaneous tissue, and muscle. Distinguishing characteristics of these entities are outlined in Table 9-2. The diagnosis of gas gangrene is usually made on clinical grounds. Local pain and swelling, severe toxemia, and muscle destruction are the typical symptoms. Jaundice, hemoglobinuria, and hemoglobinemia may be present in very severe infections, especially those involving the uterus (septic abortion). Gas is not a necessary prerequisite for diagnosis; it may be masked by extensive edema. Bacteriologic diagnosis depends upon demonstrating clostridia in the lesion, but this may reflect contamination and is meaningful only if the clinical picture is consistent with gas gangrene. A gram stain of exudate from the wound usually shows mixed bacteria and pus cells, but large gram-positive rods are the predominating organisms.

Treatment of gas gangrene includes surgery (incision, drainage, debridement, and removal of necrotic tissue), chemotherapy (antibiotics, of which penicillin is the drug of choice), and serotherapy (antitoxin—polyvalent antitoxin containing *Cl. perfringens*, *Cl. novyi*, and *Cl. septicum* antitoxins —administered systemically and locally around the wound).

Table 9-1. Toxins of **Clostridium perfringens**

Toxin	Mode of action
α	Lecithinase (lethal, dermonecrotic, hemolysin)
θ	"Hot-cold" hemolysin
κ	Collagenase
μ	Hyaluronidase
ν	Deoxyribonuclease
Others	Fibrinolysin
	Phagocytosis-inhibiting factor

Table 9-2. Differential Diagnosis of Gas Gangrene

Parameter	Gas gangrene	Anaerobic cellulitis	Streptococcal myositis
Onset	Acute	Gradual	Subacute, insidious
Toxemia	Very severe	None or slight	Severe, late
Pain	Severe	Absent	Variable, usually severe
Swelling	Marked	None or slight	Marked
Skin	Tense, white	Little change	Tense, often copper hue
Exudate	Variable, discolored (may be profuse and serous)	None or slight	Profuse (purulent or seropurulent)
Gas	Rarely pronounced	Abundant	Very slight
Odor	Variable, may be slight	Foul	Very slight
Muscle	Marked changes	No change	Edema
Incubation period	3 days	> 3 days	3–4 days

BOTULISM

Botulism is a disease resulting from the ingestion of exotoxins of *Cl. botulinum*. Six types of toxin—designated A, B, C, D, E, and F—have been identified, each requiring specific homologous antitoxin for neutralization (toxin of one type is not neutralized by the antitoxin of a heterologous type). Disease in man has been most frequently due to types A and E, occasionally to types B and F, and not to C and D. Botulinus toxins are proteins of varying molecular weight or aggregates of proteins; they are the most potent bacterial toxins known to man. Case fatality rates vary from 20% to 70% depending on the type and amount of toxin ingested. The importance of the disease is not in the number of individuals affected but in the fear that the disease may occur at all, with its potential mortality and morbidity.

Botulism generally occurs from the ingestion of food contaminated with *Cl. botulinum* spores, which germinate under specific conditions and result in production of the toxin. Proper pressure heating of food has virtually eliminated the hazard of botulism from the commercial canning industry, but sporadic outbreaks occur owing to the ingestion of improperly home-canned and preserved foods. While botulism appeared originally to be associated only with improperly preserved foods of animal origin—such as sausage, spiced meat, and fish—canned vegetables and other foods have been implicated in sporadic outbreaks of the disease. There recently was an increase in the cases of human botulism in the United States, most of them due to type E strain; surprisingly, many of the cases were traced to commercially prepared or processed foods, especially smoked whitefish vacuum-packaged in pliofilm bags. Studies stimulated by this occurrence revealed that the type E strain, like other strains of *Cl. botulinum*, resides in the soil and is probably transported to the sea via streams and surface waters; the spores of type E have been isolated from sea bottom near coastal areas and evidently are the source of contamination of fish caught for consumption.

Botulinus toxin is primarily absorbed in the stomach and upper small intestine; it is resistant to breakdown in the gastrointestinal tract, thus permitting slower absorption in the lower small intestine and colon. The toxin acts selectively on the cholinergic nerve system, sparing the adrenergic nerves. The toxin completely blocks neuromuscular transmission and acetylcholine release by interfering with nerve conduction at the terminal branches of nerve fibrils short of the motor end plate.

In most outbreaks a high proportion of persons consuming spoiled food develop clinical symptoms. Symptoms generally develop from 12 to as long as 100 hours after ingestion of toxin and include postural hypotension, ocular disturbances (diplopia, paralysis of accomodation, loss of pupillary light reflex resulting in dilated unreactive pupils), difficulty in speaking and swallowing, cessation of salivation, ileus, and paralysis of the muscles of respiration and other striated muscle groups.

Routine laboratory studies are not helpful in the diagnosis of botulism; in special studies, though, toxin has been identified in the blood of some patients with type E botulism. The presence of specific toxin is demonstrated by injecting serum from a patient into mice, which then die of an illness manifested by progressive muscular and respiratory paralysis resembling botulism; this can be prevented by the simultaneous injection of type-specific antitoxin.

Treatment consists of supportive measures, especially maintenance of an adequate airway and mechanical assistance of respiration. The administration of type-specific antitoxin may be of value; until the type of botulism is determined, administration of polyvalent antitoxin (A, B, and E) is appropriate.

SUGGESTED READING

Anaerobic Infections

1. BRAUDE AI: Anaerobic infection: diagnosis and therapy. Hosp Practice Feb: 42–46, 1968.
2. GOLDSAND G, BRAUDE AI: Anaerobic infections, Disease-A-Month. Chicago, Year Book Publishers, 1966

Tetanus

1. BULLER DH, VAUGHN CC: Clinical tetanus. Milit Med 128:867–870, 1963
2. EDSALL G, ELLIOTT MW, PEEBLES TC, et al: Excessive use of tetanus toxoid boosters. JAMA 202:17–19, 1967
3. LAFORCE FM, YOUNG LS, BENNETT JV: Tetanus in the United States (1965–1966). N Engl J Med 280:569–574, 1969
4. LEVINE L, MCCOMB JA, DWYER RC, et al: Active-passive tetanus immunization. N Engl J Med 274:186–190, 1966
5. PARSONS RL, HOFMANN WW, FEIGEN GA: Mode of tetanus toxin on the neuromuscular junction. Am J Physiol 210:84–90, 1966
6. WILLIAMS K: Some observations on Clostridium tetani. Med Lab Technol 28:399–408, 1971

Gas Gangrene

1. ALTEMEIER WA, FULLIN WD: Prevention and treatment of gas gangrene. JAMA 217:806–813, 1971
2. BAKER EE: Clostridial infections with special reference to Clostridium perfringens. Am J Surg 107:689–692, 1964

Botulism   3. MACLENNEN JD: Histotoxic clostridial infections in man. Bacteriol Rev 26:177–276, 1962

1. DOADIO JA, GANGAROSA EJ, FAICH GA: Diagnosis and treatment of botulism. J Infect Dis 124:108–112, 1971
2. ROGERS DE: Botulism, vintage 1963. Ann Intern Med 61:581–588, 1964

10

Listeria Monocytogenes

Listeria monocytogenes organisms are aerobic, short, gram-positive rods which have a tendency to appear as diplobacilli (Fig. 10-1); they appear occasionally in short chains or palisades but resemble streptococci rather than diphtheroids. The bacteriologic characteristics of the organism are outlined in Table 10-1. Although long known as a significant pathogen in animals, it has been recognized as causing disease in man only since 1929; from that time, however, it has been reported with increasing frequency, especially in persons with altered host defense mechanisms.

CLASSIFICATION The genus *Listeria* is divided into four major serologic types on the basis of somatic (O) and flagellar (H) antigens. These are designated as types 1 through 4 (1a, 1b, 2, 3a, 3b, 4a, 4b, 4c, 4ab, 4d, and 4e). Types 1, 4a, and 4b are the common serotypes producing disease in man—types 4a and 4b in the United States, type 1 in Europe.

TRANSMISSION Person to person transmission has been documented rarely, isolated cases of listeriosis being the rule. In most instances the source of infection cannot be found, although a large reservoir of infection is known to exist among animals and birds. Transmission likely occurs by means of the

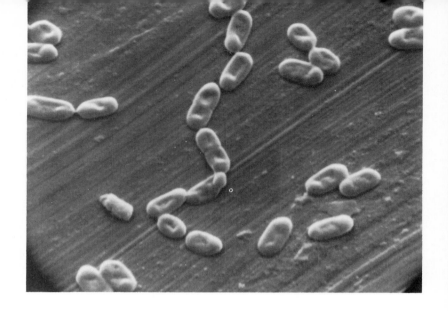

Fig. 10–1.
Listeria monocytogenes. Scanning electron micrograph demonstrating the short diplobacillary character of the organism and its occurrence in short chains. (×10,000)

Table 10-1. Bacteriologic Characteristics of Listeria monocytogenes

Short gram-positive rod
Hemolytic
Motile
Catalase-positive
Positive methyl red reactions
Acid fermentation of glucose and salicin but not mannitol
Induction of conjunctivitis when instilled into the conjunctiva of a rabbit

contamination of streams, mud, and sewage with the excreta of wild animals. Domestic animals infected via these sources probably then infect man.

DISEASE IN MAN   The following syndromes characterize human listeriosis.

Repeated Abortion

Genital listeriosis is basically a venereal disease, the father carrying the organism in the semen and prostatic secretions, the mother in vaginal fluids. This type of infection may result in repeated abortions, although the aborting mother rarely has evidence of active disease. If the chronic aborter is found to be infected and is treated, normal pregnancies then result.

Granuloma Infantisepticum

The most common form of listeriosis in infants, granuloma infantisepticum accounts for about 30% of all cases of listeriosis in humans. The fetus is probably infected by the maternal blood via the placenta and placental infection; bacteremia in the fetus results in areas of focal granulomatous necrosis in many parts of the body, especially the liver.

Meningitis and Encephalitis   About one-third of the cases of human listeriosis involve the central nervous system. Meningitis results in spinal fluid findings typical of any bacterial meningitis, although occasionally a predominance of mononuclear cells are present, some of which are atypical. Unlike most bacterial meningitides, however, the onset may be very insidious, lasting weeks or months.

Infectious Mononucleosis-like Syndrome   In some patients, listeriosis presents with fever, lymphadenopathy, splenomegaly, monocytosis with atypical cells, and a negative heterophile test. Bacteremia may be demonstrable, thus documenting the diagnosis.

Endocarditis and bacteremia also occur, the latter without other symptoms or with conjunctivitis, skin rashes, or urethritis. Recently the majority of cases seen in large medical centers are those occurring in patients with lymphoreticular diseases and those receiving corticosteroid therapy and cytotoxic agents. Premature infants, pregnant women, diabetics, and alcoholics are also prone to listeriosis.

DIAGNOSIS   Diagnosis of listeriosis is made by demonstrating the organism in the blood, spinal fluid, or other appropriate sources, and by finding a rise in the agglutination titer. It should be emphasized, however, that many apparently normal subjects have agglutinating antibodies against *L. monocytogenes*, making interpretation difficult.

SUGGESTED READING

1. GRAY ML, KILLINGER AH: Listeria monocytogenes and listeric infections. Bacteriol Rev 30:309–382, 1966
2. BUCHNER LH, SCHNEIERSON SS: Clinical and laboratory aspects of Listeria monocytogenes infections. Am J Med 45:904–920, 1968
3. BUSCH LA: Human listeriosis in the United States 1967–1969. J Infect Dis 123: 328–332, 1971
4. MEDOFF G, KUNZ LJ, WEINBERG AN: Listeriosis in humans: an evaluation. J Infect Dis 123:247–250, 1971

11

Bacillus

The genus *Bacillus* comprises many gram-positive, aerobic, sporulating rods. Except for *Bacillus anthracis*, these are generally ubiquitous, non-pathogenic saprophytes; *B. subtilis, B. megaterium, B. ramosus,* and *B. cereus* are most familiar. They are distinguished from one another by spore formation, differential fermentation, and growth characteristics on selective media. Most clinical laboratories, however, do not attempt to classify the several species but simply differentiate between *B. anthracis* and the "nonpathogenic" bacilli, the latter usually collectively classified as *B. subtilis*.

BACILLUS SUBTILIS   *B. subtilis* is a short, gram-positive rod with slightly rounded ends (Fig. 11-1). Although spores are generally not clearly visible, one occasionally sees slight swelling of the middle of the organism without much distortion of cell outline. The organism has a characteristic sluggish, twisting type of motility described as "swarming." It is commonly found in dust and hay (the "hay bacillus"). When isolated from clinical material, even blood or cerebrospinal fluid, it has generally been considered a contaminant. However, this organism may cause localized or disseminated infection.

Infection of the eye is most common after ocular trauma (e.g., presence of a foreign body, penetrating injury of the globe, surgical procedures) and may involve any portion of the eye or its surrounding structures. Infection after ophthalmic surgery may be related to the high resistance of the spores to chemical disinfectants used in sterilizing surgical instruments.

Fig. 11–1.
Bacillus subtilis. Scanning electron micrograph demonstrating the typical rod-shaped appearance with slightly rounded ends. A naked cell wall is seen in the middle of the field. (×10,000)

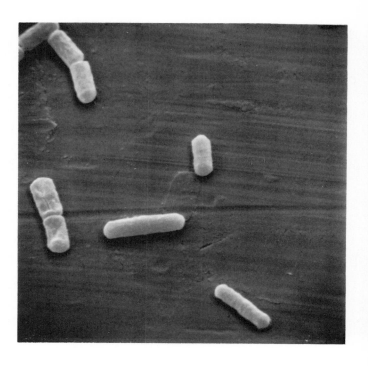

The organism has been implicated in pneumonia, lung abscess, pleuritis, peritonitis, and pericarditis. *B. subtilis* pyelonephritis, cystitis, and prostatitis have also been described, usually as complications of bladder catheterization.

B. subtilis may cause abscess formation and cellulitis of the skin, the most fulminating example being postoperative cellulitis, generally of the abdominal wall. This disorder is due to synergistic infection with an anaerobic streptococcus.

Disseminated infection via the bloodstream usually involves the central nervous system and may present as meningitis, myelitis, or encephalitis. Meningitis may complicate mastoiditis, otitis media, or the administration of spinal anesthesia. *B. subtilis* bacteremia may also result in endocarditis, with infection generally occurring on a previously damaged heart valve.

ANTHRAX   *Bacillus anthracis* is a large, spore-forming, gram-positive rod which may be arranged in chains. The exact mechanism by which the organism causes disease is not entirely clear, but the anthrax bacillus is known to produce a lethal toxin which alters the body's physiology primarily via the central nervous system and kills by terminal anoxia mediated by the central nervous system.

Essentially anthrax is a disease of animals; it accidentally becomes an industrial disease of man. Anthrax spores can survive for years, so that both in space and time human infection may be widely separated from the animal from which it came. An animal dying of anthrax in Argentina may have parts of its carcass distributed into a wide variety of industries in many parts of the world and thereby expose workers in the wool, felt, horsehair, brush, and bristle industries, as well as those that utilize the animal's hide, skin, and bone. In general, then, two classes of workers may become infected: 1) those who handle the animal or its dead carcass, and 2) those who later handle parts of the carcass. The former include cattlemen, goat herds, veterinarians, and butchers; the latter, dock workers who take part in transporting infected materials, tannery workers (leather workers rarely become infected because the tanning process usually destroys the organism), upholsterers, carpet workers, workers in the clothing industry exposed to wool and hair, and persons in the glue and fertilizer industries exposed to bones and hooves.

The incubation period of the disease is 2 or 3 days, after which one of three clinical forms of the disease appears.

Cutaneous Anthrax

Cutaneous anthrax presents as a malignant pustule, the commonest form of the disease. It starts as a tiny pimple, which then enlarges in 1–3 days, developing a ring of blisters; at first these are clear and glistening, but later they become bluish and full of blood. The central pimple ulcerates and rapidly dries to form a central scab. This firmly adhering black scab and the surrounding bluish vesicles comprise the malignant pustule, which almost always is surrounded by severe edema. (If the malignant pustule is on an extremity, the entire limb may be swollen; if on the forehead, the eyes may be closed and the whole face swollen; and if on the neck, the swelling may cause respiratory embarrassment by pressing on the trachea.) No matter how red, swollen, and hot the affected part may be, however, there is rarely any pus. Local lymphadenitis is common but is not usually severe or painful; in fact, pain is not a prominent symptom in anthrax, although the pustule and the edema may appear extremely tender. The degree of systemic symptoms varies; nausea, headache, and chilliness are common; fever is usually low-grade. In severe cases, high fever (greater than 103°F), vomiting, prostration, and shock are ominous signs. The fatality rate is about 5%. In treated patients symptoms subside in a few days, but the pustule takes 2–3 weeks to heal. Organisms are demonstrable only during the first 2 days after treatment so that isolation of the patient need not be maintained until the pustule heals.

Pulmonary Anthrax

"Woolsorters' disease" is a fulminating form of pulmonary anthrax with sudden onset, high fever, shaking chills, and respiratory distress. Untreated, the disease is almost always fatal. The patient's occupation is the clue to the diagnosis.

Intestinal Anthrax

Intestinal anthrax presents as severe enteritis and is caused by eating infected meat.

The diagnosis of anthrax in the cutaneous form is simple if the patient's occupation is known and the possibility of anthrax is considered. A gram stain of the lesion is almost diagnostic and can be substantiated by culture.

SUGGESTED READING

1. FARRAR WE JR: Serious infections due to "non-pathogenic" organisms of the genus Bacillus. Am J Med 34:134–141, 1963
2. CHRISTIE AB: Anthrax. Practitioner 191:588–593, 1963

12

Hemophilus

The genus *Hemophilus* is composed of a heterogeneous group of aerobic, nonmotile, nonspore-forming, small, gram-negative rods that for growth require enriched media usually containing blood or blood products. Some members of the genus are part of the normal flora of the mucous membranes, whereas others such as *Hemophilus influenzae* are important human pathogens and can result in otitis media, meningitis, pneumonia, endocarditis, and arthritis.

HEMOPHILUS INFLUENZAE

Typically these organisms are small, pleomorphic, encapsulated coccobacilli; filamentous and large spherical forms also occur, cultural morphology varying with age and growth medium (Fig. 12-1). On chocolate agar (containing heated blood), the most commonly employed medium for the isolation and identification of this organism, colonies are small (1–2 mm in diameter) and transparent; around staphylococci, colonies grow much larger (satellite phenomenon). *H. influenzae* requires growth factors X (hemin) and V (probably coenzyme I or II or nicotinamide nucleoside; growth in symbiosis with staphylococci, which produce V factor, is the basis for the satellite phenomenon). Members of the *Hemophilus* genus are identified in part by differential needs for X and V factors (Table 12-1).

H. influenzae is classified by type-specific capsular polysaccharides into six types: a, b, c, d, e, and f. The capsular polysaccharides of *H. influenzae*

Fig. 12–1.
Scanning electron micrograph of
Hemophilus influenzae demonstrating
the pleomorphic morphology of the
bacillus. (×10,000)

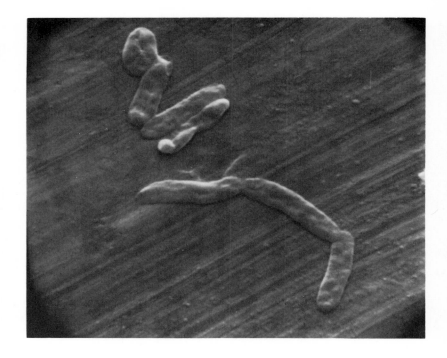

Table 12-1. Differential Growth Requirements
of the Genus Hemophilus

Organism	Requires X	V
H. influenzae	+	+
H. parainfluenzae	−	+
H. hemolyticus	+	+
Bordetella pertussis	−	−

are similar to the specific soluble substances of pneumococci; therefore, cross reactions may occur with certain types of pneumococci. The quellung reaction can be used to type *H. influenzae.*

Although nonencapsulated organisms are part of the normal flora of the respiratory tract of man, encapsulated forms can produce suppurative disease. The pathogenesis of *H. influenzae* infections is not well understood. The organism produces no exotoxin; endotoxins can be demonstrated, although their role in producing diseases is uncertain.

Meningitis

Hemophilus influenzae meningitis, most often due to type b *H. influenzae,* is most common in children, with a peak incidence between the ages of 6 months and 3 years. It presents as a typical bacterial meningitis with the usual spinal fluid findings; a gram stain of the spinal fluid reveals pleomorphic gram-negative coccobacilli frequently with bipolar, more deeply staining granules. Sterile subdural effusions are a common complication and one of the reasons for the morbidity of the disease.

Otitis Media

H. influenzae is a common cause of suppurative otitis media in children.

Epiglottitis

Epiglottitis of bacterial origin is most often due to *H. influenzae* and can result in airway occlusion and death due to asphyxia. Downward spread results in laryngitis, tracheitis, and bronchitis, all of which may cause respiratory embarrassment. Exacerbations of chronic bronchitis in persons with chronic obstructive bronchopulmonary disease is felt to be incited by or due to *H. influenzae* infection. Pneumonia, endocarditis, pericarditis, genitourinary tract infection, suppurative arthritis, cellulitis, and osteomyelitis due to *H. influenzae* have also been reported.

It was previously thought that acute *H. influenzae* infections occurred only during childhood because after the age of 3 years there was widespread development of bactericidal antibody. However, an increasing number of infections are being seen in adults, with a parallel demonstration of an increasing number of nonimmune individuals beyond childhood. Whether this phenomenon is due to early treatment of *H. influenzae* infections in childhood with antibiotics is not known.

OTHER HEMOPHILUS SPECIES OF SIGNIFICANCE

H. aegypticus. Also known as the Koch-Weeks bacillus, this is the cause of epidemic purulent conjunctivitis during the summer months.

H. ducreyi. This is the etiologic agent of chancroid, a venereal disease characterized by a swollen, tender, ragged ulcer on the genitalia and enlarged, painful local lymphadenopathy. Smears of the lesion demonstrate small gram-negative rods in strands. Suspensions of killed *H. ducreyi* are useful as a skin test antigen for the diagnosis of chancroid (Ducrey's skin test); the test becomes positive 1–2 weeks after infection.

WHOOPING COUGH

The clinical entity whooping cough is caused by *Bordetella pertussis*, a short, gram-negative coccobacillus resembling but less pleomorphic than *H. influenzae*. The whooping cough bacillus is included here because of its previous classification in the genus *Hemophilus*; *Bordetella* is a newly created genus which includes *B. pertussis*, *B. parapertussis*, and *B. bronchiseptica*.

Optimum isolation of *B. pertussis* requires complex, enriched media, the most common of which is Bordet-Gengou's medium (potato-blood-glycerol-agar); the organism also grows on blood agar with a narrow zone of hemolysis. Variations in growth phases are listed in Table 12-2.

B. pertussis is an obligate parasite transmitted via droplet from man to man, the patient in the catarrhal stage of the disease or with subclinical disease being the major source. The organism multiplies rapidly in the mucous membranes of the respiratory tract and invades by continuity to

Table 12-2. Variations in Growth Phases of Bordetella pertussis

Phase	Colonial morphology	Virulence
I	Smooth (encapsulated)	Virulent
II	Smooth—rough	Intermediate
III	Rough—smooth	Intermediate
IV	Rough (nonencapsulated)	Avirulent

involve all layers of the respiratory epithelium. Bloodstream invasion is rare.

The incubation period of whooping cough is approximately 2 weeks. The first symptom of the disease is a cough, but sneezing is not uncommon during the early or catarrhal stage. During the catarrhal stage, which lasts about a week, the patient may not be very ill but is highly infectious because of the large number of organisms sprayed in droplets. During the spasmodic or paroxysmal stage, the typical expiratory cough develops characterized by a staccato rhythm during which paroxysms of coughing get closer and closer and faster and faster; at the end of each episode the patient drools ropy, foamy mucus, may vomit, and then draws air back into the lungs with a loud whoop. Several episodes of coughing may occur at a time or the patient may appear entirely well—even sleep—between paroxysms. Episodes of coughing may be severe enough to result in cyanosis, convulsions, and coma. Low-grade fever may accompany the disease, but high fever usually signifies secondary bacterial infection (otitis media, pneumonia with *Staphylococcus aureus, Streptococcus pyogenes, Diplococcus pneumoniae* or *Hemophilus influenzae*). The disease usually lasts 4–6 weeks, and during this time other complications may occur: severe malnutrition, dehydration, atelectasis secondary to airway obstruction by mucous plugs, and hernias.

The diagnosis of whooping cough is made on the basis of the clinical picture and is documented by culture. The organism is most easily demonstrated during the catarrhal stage of the disease and thereafter with decreasing frequency. Cough plates or nasopharyngeal cultures are most useful.

Control of whooping cough depends on early diagnosis, isolation of cases, and immunization. Pertussis vaccine—usually given as DPT (diphtheria, pertussis, tetanus vaccine)—consists of killed phase I organisms; three injections are given during the first year of life with boosters a year later and after known exposure. Persons exposed to whooping cough without prior immunization may be given hyperimmune γ-globulin for temporary passive protection.

The whooping cough syndrome has been attributed to adenoviruses and some other respiratory pathogens such as B. *parapertussis* and B. *bronchiseptica*, emphasizing that all children with cough and whooping do not have whooping cough, and all children with pertussis do not whoop.

SUGGESTED READING

1. ALEXANDER HE: The hemophilus group, Bacterial and Mycotic Infections of Man. Fourth edition. Edited by RJ Dubos and JG Hirsch. Philadelphia, Lippincott, 1965, p 724

2. BRADFORD WL: The bordetella group, Bacterial and Mycotic Infections of Man. Fourth edition. Edited by RJ Dubos and JG Hirsch. Philadelphia, Lippincott, 1965, p 742

3. CONNOR JD: Evidence for an etiologic role of adenoviral infection in pertussis syndrome. N Engl J Med 283:390–394, 1970

4. KENDRICK PL: Guest editorial. Health Lab Sci 8:194–196, 1971

13

Enteric Gram-Negative Bacilli

The enteric organism comprising the family Enterobacteriaceae are a heterogeneous but interrelated group of aerobic, nonsporeforming, relatively straight, gram-negative rods with rounded ends. They are variously motile. Some are encapsulated. All ferment glucose with or without gas formation. Their natural habitat is the intestinal tract of man, but some can cause significant disease, e.g., pneumonia and urinary tract infection when they occur elsewhere; salmonellae and shigellae are the causative agents of intestinal infections.

Although it is not the purpose of this text to discuss the laboratory identification of each of the several genera and many species, Figure 13-1 is included merely as an outline of simple differentiation of the enteric organisms of medical significance. It should be emphasized that separation into the lactose fermenters and nonlactose fermenters is merely a useful method of gross classification, the four nonlactose fermenters—*Salmonella*, *Shigella*, *Proteus*, and *Pseudomonas*—can thus be distinguished from the remainder of the group.

COLIFORM BACTERIA   The coliform group includes *Escherichia*, *Aerobacter*, *Klebsiella*, and the paracolon bacilli. Morphologically they are similar (Figs. 13-2 through 13-4), but they are antigenically complex and manifest variable serologic behavior. They are classified by heat-stable somatic (O) antigens, heat-labile capsular (K) antigens, and flagellar (H) antigens. Klebsiella possess

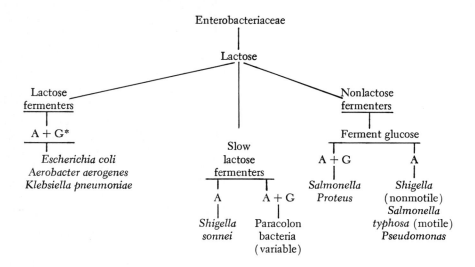

Fig. 13–1.
Gross differentiation of the Enterobacteriaceae. *A: ferment lactose (glucose) with the production of acid. A+G: ferment lactose (glucose) with the production of acid and gas.

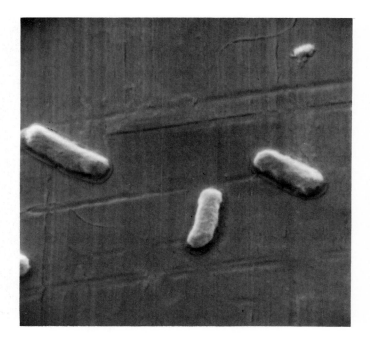

Fig. 13–2.
Escherichia coli. Scanning electron micrograph demonstrating typical appearance of gram-negative enteric bacilli. Although some differences in the morphology of the enteric bacilli may be seen, none are so characteristic as to allow absolute differentiation on morphologic grounds alone. (×10,000)

large polysaccharide capsules and can be identified by capsular swelling tests. The coliforms make up a large part of the intestinal flora of man but can play the role of significant pathogens when they invade tissues outside the gastrointestinal tract, especially the lungs, genitourinary tract, hepatobiliary tract, peritoneum, or meninges. They also may cause disease in the host with altered defense mechanisms. Two entities which deserve special mention are urinary tract infection and *Klebsiella* pneumonia.

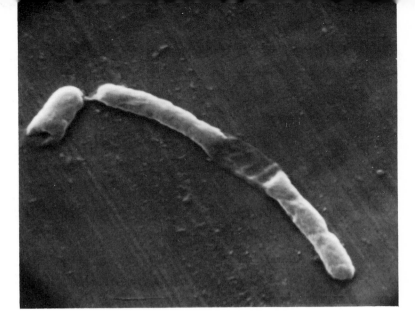

Fig. 13–3.
Aerobacter aerogenes: scanning electron micrograph. (×10,000)

Fig. 13–4.
Klebsiella pneumoniae. Scanning electron micrograph demonstrating mucoid appearance and part of the capsule. (×10,000)

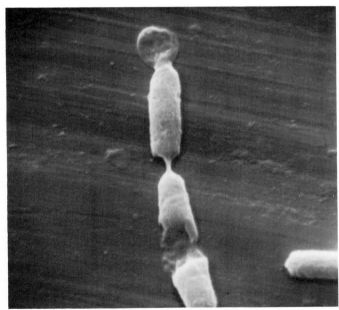

Urinary Tract Infection   Urinary tract infections include a spectrum of familiar clinical entities in which the presence of bacteriuria is the common denominator. Under the age of 1 year the prevalence of bacteriuria is 1–2% in both males and females and is frequently associated with the presence of congenital structural abnormalities of the genitourinary tract. In the female the occurrence of bacteriuria remains stable at the same rate through childhood but increases by 1% per decade thereafter. By the age of 50 years the prevalence is approximately 10%. In the male, bacteriuria is distinctly uncommon after the first year of life; by middle age, however, the incidence of prostatic, bladder, and urethral disease rises rapidly, and elderly males have the same incidence of bacteriuria as their female counterparts. The greater prevalence of bacteriuria in females between the ages of 1 and 50 years is probably related to anatomic differences between the sexes. In both cases the distal urethra is normally contaminated with skin and fecal flora. Because the female urethra is shorter, however, ascent of bacteria to the bladder is more easily accomplished. In addition, urinary tract infections seem to occur more commonly in relationship to sexual activity and childbirth, which are associated with urethral trauma. Statistical studies designed to confirm this relationship, however, have been inconclusive.

While urinary tract infections may occasionally result from hematogenous spread of bacteria from distant foci or via lymphatics from the lower gastrointestinal and genitourinary tracts, the vast majority result from the intraluminal ascent of bacteria through the urethra to the bladder and then potentially to the renal medulla via the ureter. While urine is an excellent culture medium, the normal voiding mechanism and the presence of certain poorly defined antibacterial factors in the bladder mucosa inhibit the ascent of bacteria to the bladder and are usually capable of eliminating bladder colonization if it occurs. Interference with these natural defenses result in a greater likelihood of bacterial ascent and multiplication, which may then evoke an inflammatory response and symptomatic disease. Factors which interfere with normal defenses include obstruction and stasis, which may result from either functional or anatomic variances such as strictures, prostatic hypertrophy, congenital abnormalities, neurologic abnormalities, etc. Foreign bodies and residua of previous inflammatory diseases such as stones, debris, and mucus may also enhance susceptibility. Once bacteria colonize the bladder there is an open system which provides for ascent to the renal medulla. Ascent may be facilitated by the presence of vesicoureteral reflux. In addition, the renal medulla is particularly susceptible to infection; the hypertonic environment antagonizes phagocytosis and perhaps provides a favorable environment for the survival of bacteria in spite of natural defenses and antimicrobial therapy. The presence of certain systemic conditions such as hypertension, diabetes mellitus, gout, hypokalemia, hypercalcemia, nephrocalcinosis, and nephrolithiasis are known to increase further the susceptibility of the renal parenchyma to infection. Thus the acquisition of bacteriuria requires the ascent of bacteria to and their subsequent multiplication in the bladder.

Irrespective of clinical presentation, urinalysis, or radiographic or anatomic findings, examination of the urine for bacteria is the most direct and reliable means of diagnosing a urinary tract infection. The usual method for diagnosing bacteriuria is by quantitative culture of a urine specimen obtained by the clean-catch midstream technique. A fixed volume (usually 0.01 ml) of urine is then inoculated on agar plates, the number of colonies counted, and the number of colony-forming units (bacteria) in the original specimen then calculated. Colony counts of 10^5 or greater are considered to represent "significant bacteriuria," since the majority of patients with urinary tract infections have this many bacteria in each milliliter of their urine. Colony counts of 10^4 or less are considered to be "insignificant," since contamination, frequently with multiple skin or mucosal inhabitants, may result in a lesser degree of growth. Results of urine cultures and colony counts can be obtained only after 24 hours. The presence of 10 to 15 or more bacteria per high power field of spun urinary sediment or the presence of any bacteria in a gram-stained drop of unspun urine correlate fairly well with colony counts of 10^5 or greater and may be used to establish the diagnosis of "significant bacteriuria" in a patient in whom waiting 24 hours or longer to start treatment is inadvisable. The urinalysis provides additional information in that leukocytes (sometimes in clumps or casts), erythrocytes, and/or protein may be present with infection. These findings by themselves are not diagnostic of bacteriuria, however, since they may be present in persons with chronic renal disease, nonbacterial genitourinary disease, and many systemic diseases.

Escherichia coli is the pathogen in approximately 90% of acute uncomplicated urinary tract infections. *Proteus mirabilis*, klebsiella, enterobacter, staphylococci, or enterococci are occasionally responsible. In patients who have had repeated infections, underlying genitourinary or systemic disease, structural abnormalities, instrumentation, or in whom infection is hospital-acquired, the etiologic agents are more varied and more likely to be resistant to multiple antibiotics. Under these circumstances, *E. coli* is still most common (50%). Other pathogens include *P. mirabilis* (20%), klebsiella, enterobacter, pseudomonas, mixed organisms, enterococci, staphylococci, and others (about 5% each). The gram-positive cocci are most frequently isolated from elderly males with prostatic disease. Selection of therapy must be based upon consideration of 1) the severity and extent of the clinical illness, 2) the etiologic agent and its antimicrobial sensitivities, and 3) the underlying conditions of the patient.

Special problems encountered with urinary tract infection include the following.

School Screening. Routine screening of healthy school girls has revealed a prevalence of 1–2% asymptomatic bacteriuria. A population "at risk" for the development of symptomatic disease and possible renal damage can therefore be identified and treated.

Pregnancy. The prevalence of asymptomatic bacteriuria in pregnant women is approximately 6%. Among this group 40% develop acute pyelonephritis, and 50% have abnormal intravenous pyelograms. Premature delivery, perinatal infant death, and preeclampsia occur with a higher frequency than in nonbacteriuric pregnant females, and as a group the bacteriuric women have statistically higher blood urea nitrogen values and decreased urine concentrating ability. Treatment of bacteriuria lowers the incidence of acute pyelonephritis but may not reduce the incidence of other complications. Follow-up is imperative, since recurrence of bacteriuria later in pregnancy or post partum occurs in many cases.

Diabetes Mellitus. While the metabolic defect in diabetes may not predispose to bacteriuria, diabetics are more likely to have neurologic bladder dysfunction, structural renal disease, instrumentation, frequent hospitalization—and therefore a higher incidence of urinary tract infection. Keto-acidosis does result in increased susceptibility to infection.

Bladder Catheterization. Simple insertion and removal of a catheter, even with careful technique, results in a 1–2% infection rate. An indwelling catheter, which remains in the bladder, results in an infection rate that rises with time; by 4 to 5 days the prevalence of infection is approximately 95%.

Reflux. Reflux of urine from the bladder to the ureter and subsequently to the kidney is frequently associated with urinary tract infections in children. Its presence may be the result of infection, bladder outlet obstruction, or abnormalities of the ureterovesicle junction.

Klebsiella Pneumonia   About 2% of all bacterial pneumonias are due to infection with *Klebsiella pneumoniae*. This results in hemorrhagic consolidation of the lungs, which may progress to microabscess formation and fibrosis unless properly treated. In alcoholics there is an increased frequency of upper lobe pneumonia due to this organism.

PROTEUS   Proteus organisms are nonlactose-fermenting, motile, aerobic, gram-negative rods which tend to "swarm" or spread rapidly over the surface of solid media (Fig. 13-5). They are a not uncommon cause of urinary tract infections or other disease in altered hosts. In this regard, division into indole-positive and indole-negative groups is of clinical importance because the former organisms (*P. vulgaris, P. morgani, P. rettgeri*) are difficult to treat, whereas the latter (*P. mirabilis*) are usually sensitive to large doses of penicillin or ampicillin. About 60–70% of proteus infections, especially of the urinary tract, are due to indole-negative strains.

PSEUDOMONAS   The pseudomonas group of organisms, of which *Pseudomonas aeruginosa* is the prototype (Fig. 13-6), are gram-negative, motile rods; they produce water-soluble pigments, pyocyanin and fluorescein, which endow colonies on solid culture media with a fluorescent greenish color. Some strains are hemolytic. Pseudomonas organisms make up only a small part of the normal intestinal flora of man, but they are becoming pathogens of increasing importance in patients with altered host defense mechanisms.

SALMONELLA   The salmonellae are gram-negative, motile rods (Fig. 13-7) which do not ferment lactose and are pathogenic for man via the oral route. They are identified by biochemical reactions and antigenic characteristics. There are three main species—*Salmonella enteritidis*, *S. typhi*, and *S. choleraesuis*—which are subclassified into bioserotypes (biochemically and serologically different) and serotypes (biochemically similar and serologically different). There are three main antigens: somatic "O" antigens designated

Fig. 13–5.
Proteus vulgaris. Multiple flagella are evident as is the leaf-like ellipsoidal appearance of the gram-negative bacilli due to osmotic changes in the environment (in this case 15% sucrose). (Klainer AS, Betsch CJ: J Infect Dis 121:339–343, Copyright [1970] The University of Chicago) (×10,000)

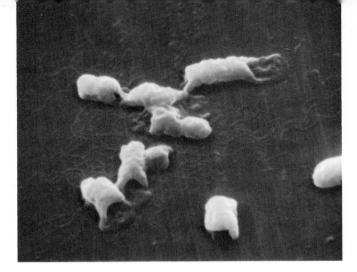

Fig. 13–6.
Pseudomonas aeruginosa: Scanning electron micrograph. (Klainer AS, Perkins RL: J Infect Dis 122:323–328, Copyright [1970] The University of Chicago) (×10,000)

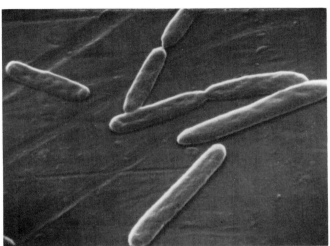

Fig. 13–7.
Salmonella species: Scanning electron micrograph. (×10,000)

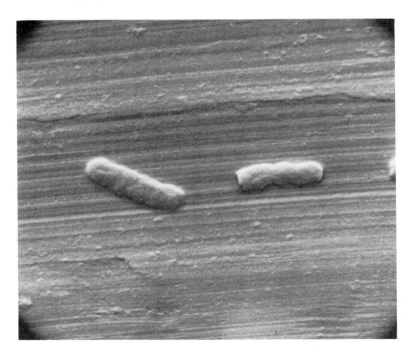

Table 13-1. Speciation of Salmonellae (Older Classification)

Group A:	*S. paratyphosa* (paratyphoid A)
Group B:	*S. schottmuelleri* (paratyphoid B), *S. typhimurium*
Group C₁:	*S. hirschfeldii* (paratyphoid C), *S. oranienberg*, *S. montevideo*, *S. choleraesuis*
Group C₂:	*S. newporti*
Group D:	*S. typhosa*, *S. enteritidis*, *S. gallinarum—pullorum*
Group E:	*S. anatum*

by Roman numerals, flagellar "H" antigens designated by small letters and small numbers, and the "Vi" antigen thought to be related to virulence. Thus antigenic constitution might be described as *S. typhosa* 9, 12, Vi, d. Although this is the most recent classification, the older method of speciation is sufficiently familiar to warrant mention (Table 13-1).

There are four major kinds of salmonella infection: 1) gastroenteritis, 2) the enteric fevers, 3) the bacteremias, and 4) the carrier state.

Gastroenteritis

Gastroenteritis is the most common clinical illness caused by the salmonellae. Infection is via ingestion of food contaminated by a carrier. As the food sits the organism multiplies; the severity of subsequent disease is usually related to the number of viable organisms ingested. In gastroenteritis, infection is limited to the mucosa of the gastrointestinal tract; bacteremia is uncommon except in young infants, the elderly, and patients with underlying debilitating disease. The organisms most commonly implicated in gastroenteritis are *S. choleraesuis* and *S. enteritidis* serotypes *typhimurium, montivideo,* and *newport.* In the United States *S. enteritidis* serotype *typhimurium* is most common. The incubation period of the disease is 24–48 hours. The illness is characterized by nausea, vomiting, diarrhea, and abdominal pain of varying intensity. Diarrhea may be bloody. Systemic reaction, i.e., fever, is variable. The disease usually lasts less than a week and is generally self-limited. Diagnosis is made by demonstrating the organism in the stool; a gram stain of the stool shows pus cells.

Enteric Fevers

The enteric fevers are basically diseases of lymphoid tissue. The pathogenesis of the enteric fevers is outlined in Figure 13-8. The prototype of the enteric fevers is typhoid fever. Diarrhea occurs in only 60–70% of those who have an enteric fever, constipation being a common presenting symptom. The clinical picture is characterized by fever, bradycardia, hepatosplenomegaly, and leukopenia. Some patients manifest "rose spots," fleeting pink macular lesions on the anterior abdominal wall which may harbor organisms. The diagnosis is made by demonstrating the organism in the blood (first week of the disease), stool (second week), and urine (third week). Metastatic infection via bacteremia may occur. The three major complications are gastrointestinal hemorrhage, perforation, and relapse.

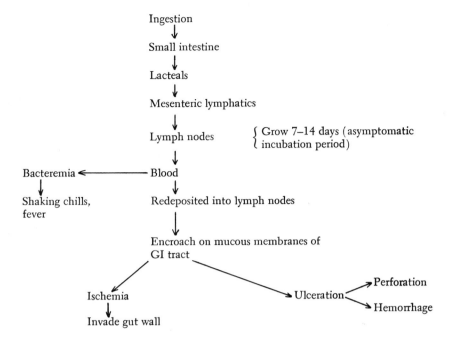

Fig. 13–8.
Pathogenesis of the enteric fevers.

Ingestion
↓
Small intestine
↓
Lacteals
↓
Mesenteric lymphatics
↓
Lymph nodes   { Grow 7–14 days (asymptomatic incubation period)
↓
Bacteremia ← Blood
↓   ↓
Shaking chills, fever   Redeposited into lymph nodes
↓
Encroach on mucous membranes of GI tract
↙   ↘
Ischemia   Ulceration → Perforation
↓   → Hemorrhage
Invade gut wall

Bacteremia   A primary focus of infection is rarely found in salmonella bacteremia. *S. choleraesuis* is the most common organism implicated. The disease usually presents as a fever of obscure etiology, the diagnosis made by demonstrating the organism in the blood. Metastatic infection is frequent —more so than in the enteric fevers—the meninges, lungs, joints, and bone being the most common sites. The salmonella bacteremias occur mainly in patients with underlying predisposing factors (Table 13-2). Most deaths due to salmonella infections occur from the bacteremias.

Table 13-2. Factors Predisposing to Salmonella Bacteremia

Old age, especially males
Cirrhosis of the liver
Cancer, especially neuroblastoma and carcinoma of the colon
Sickle cell anemia
Malaria
Louse-borne relapsing fever
Orroya fever (bartonellosis), especially during the hemolytic phase
Abdominal aortic aneurysm
Artificial cardiac valves
Antibiotic and corticosteroid therapy

Carrier State   About 0.2% of persons in the United States are salmonella carriers. There are three types of carriers: 1) permanent carriers (uncommon) who probably carry the organism in the biliary tract, 2) convalescent carriers who may carry it for 1–6 months following salmonella infection and then generally cease spontaneously, and 3) transient carriers.

Prevention of salmonella infections depends to a great degree on adequate sanitary measures as well as identifying carriers and preventing them from handling food. Recently, commercially processed poultry was identified as a major source of salmonellae, a problem which needs attention. A variety of vaccines are available consisting of killed bacterial suspensions of several salmonella types, especially *S. typhi*; at present these are administered parenterally, but oral vaccines are being investigated. Available vaccines are of questionable efficacy and probably protect against minor but not major exposures.

SHIGELLA Shigellae (Fig. 13-9) are nonmotile, aerobic, gram-negative rods which do not ferment lactose (except for *Shigella sonnei*, which is a slow lactose fermenter). Shigellae have a complex antigenic structure with much cross reaction between different species and other enteric bacteria. The principal pathogenic species are *S. shiga* (*dysenteriae*), which is rare in the United States; *S. flexneri* (*paradysenteriae*); *S. boydii*; and *S. sonnei. S. sonnei* and *S. flexneri* are the most common organisms encountered in the United States. Some shigellae are typed by colicin production. (Colicins are naturally occurring antibiotics produced by many members of the Enterobacteriaceae.)

The major importance of the shigellae is their role as the etiologic agent of bacillary dysentery, the most common of the bacterial diarrheas. Bacillary dysentery is basically a disease of the colon (occasionally the

Fig. 13–9.
Shigella sonnei: Scanning electron micrograph. (×10,000)

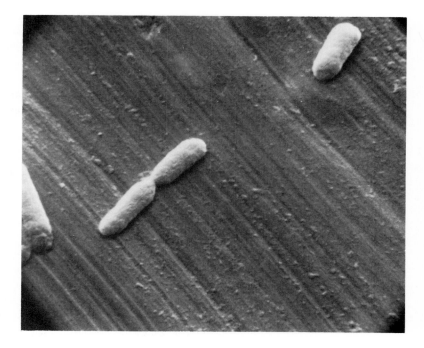

Table 13-3. *Differential Features of Common Infectious Diarrheas*

Etiology	Symptoms	Features	Laboratory findings
Viral gastroenteritis	Fever, usually low-grade or absent	Summer prevalence, ± rash	No pus cells in stool; enteroviruses may be demonstrated
Shigellosis	Abdominal pain, fever, diarrhea	Incub 1–5 days, abrupt onset, lasts 7–15 days	Stool culture; pus cells in stool
Salmonella enteritis	Diarrhea, fever, abdominal pain	Incub 8–24 hours, lasts 2–7 days	Stools positive in 50–85%; pus cells in stools
Staphylococcal food poisoning	Vomiting	Incub 4–12 hours, lasts less than 24 hours, pertinent history of food ingestion	Recovery of toxin-producing staphylococci from food
Staphylococcal enterocolitis	Fulminant diarrhea, fever	After oral antibiotics, abdominal surgery	Stool smear showing predominantly gram-positive cocci and pus cells
Amebic colitis	Diarrhea, abdominal pain, may have no fever	Gradual onset	Trophozoites and mononuclear cells in stool

terminal ileum is involved); bloodstream invasion is rare. The incubation period is 1–5 days. The illness is characterized by fever, abdominal pain, diarrhea (usually bloody, explosive, and accompanied by tenesmus). The dangers of shigellosis are water and electrolyte loss and subsequent circulatory collapse and shock. Diagnosis is made by demonstrating the organism in the stool; a gram stain of the stool shows pus cells. Bacillary dysentery frequently must be differentiated from other infectious diarrheas; Table 13-3 outlines the differential features of the common types of acute infectious diarrhea.

Shigellae are transmitted from man to man by food, fingers, feces, and flies. Good sanitation and preventing carriers from handling food are the keys to controlling shigellosis.

VIBRIOS

Cholera

Vibrios are curved, comma-shaped, aerobic, gram-negative rods which are motile and possess a single polar flagellum. *Vibrio comma (cholerae)* produces cholera in man.

Cholera is an acute diarrheal illness with an incubation period of 2 to 5 days. It is characterized by the sudden onset of nausea, vomiting, abdominal cramps, and diarrhea productive of voluminous amounts of watery stool resembling "rice water" and containing mucus, epithelial cells, and large numbers of V. comma. There is an acute loss of fluid and electrolytes with subsequent severe dehydration, vascular collapse, and shock. Cholera is rare in the United States but is not uncommon in underdeveloped countries. El Tor vibrios cause a milder diarrheal illness.

SERRATIA
(CHROMOBACTERIA)

Chromobacteria are nonsporulating, aerobic, actively motile, gram-negative rods which produce pigment on solid media in the presence of oxygen. Pigment production is most abundant on primary culture; the pigments are generally water-insoluble. *Serratia marcescens* (*Chromobacterium prodigiosum*) produces a bright red or pink pigment, C. *violaceum* a violet pigment, and C. *aquatalis* a yellow, yellow-blue, or orange pigment. These organisms are classified as Enterobacteriaceae. They are ordinarily saprophytic. In the external environment they are found in soil, water, and sewage; in man they are natural inhabitants of the bowel, lower urinary tract, and skin. They have been used as markers because their pigment can be used to study controlled infection. For example, S. *marcescens* has been applied to teeth and gums before extraction to demonstrate subsequent bacteremia; it has also been used in aerosols to study mechanisms of pulmonary infection.

The genitourinary tract is the most common site of disease. Infection almost always occurs after catheterization or treatment with multiple antibiotics; etiology is easily established by culture. Urinary tract infection may proceed to septicemia, endocarditis, and pneumonia.

The respiratory tract is also a common site of infection. Equipment used for bronchial toilet and ventilatory assistance may be a source of infection here.

Bacteremia is usually a complication of a serious or debilitating illness and is characterized by either a fulminating or chronic course. S. *marcescens* is a common contaminant of burns and surgical wounds. It has been implicated in meningitis following lumbar puncture, as well as in otitis media, sinusitis, osteomyelitis, and infantile diarrhea.

The nonchromogenic species of *Serratia* cause disease more frequently than was previously realized; perhaps they were missed because of the difficulty encountered in identifying them. Bacteremia, urinary tract infection, respiratory tract infection, osteomyelitis, and postoperative wound infection due to nonchromogenic variants of S. *marcescens* have been reported. Because of their lack of pigment production, these organisms are usually incorrectly identified as aerobacter or paracolon bacteria. The enterobacter-klebsiella-serratia group of organisms is rapidly emerging as a major cause of nosocomial infections and deserves careful watching.

Since many strains of chromobacteria are resistant to the commonly used antibiotics, therapy should be dictated by sensitivity studies. The fatality rate is high, however, even in many cases treated with antibiotics to which the organisms are sensitive by *in vitro* testing.

SUGGESTED READING

1. BLACK PH, KUNZ LG, SWARTZ MN: Salmonellosis: a review of some unusual aspects. N Engl J Med 262:811–817, 864–870, 921–927, 1960

2. MAGNUSON CW, ELSTON HR: Infections caused by nonpigmented Serratia. Ann Intern Med 65:409–418, 1966

3. MORGAN HR: The enteric bacteria, Bacterial and Mycotic Infections of Man. Fourth edition. Edited by RJ Dubos and JG Hirsch. Philadelphia, Lippincott, 1965, p. 610

4. SANDERS CV, LUBY JP, JOHANSON WG, et al: Serratia marcescens infections from inhalation therapy medications: nosocomial outbreak. Ann Intern Med 73:15–21, 1970

5. SOPHRA I, WINTER JW: Clinical manifestations of salmonellosis in man. N Engl J Med 256:1128–1134, 1957

6. WEINSTEIN L: The Practice of Infectious Disease. New York, Landsberger Medical Books, 1958, pp. 243–268

7. WILFERT JN, BARRETT FF, KASS EH: Bacteremia due to Serratia marcescens. N Engl J Med 279:286–289, 1968

14

Bacteroides

The bacteroides (Fig. 14-1) constitute a large group of nonsporeforming, strictly anaerobic, nonmotile, usually gram-negative, pleomorphic bacteria; they inhabit all mucous membranes but are most numerous in the lower intestine and are considered to be the predominant organism in human feces. Many species of *Bacteroides* grow in simple media such as peptone water, but there is wide variation in growth requirements. Isolation is most successful in media enriched with blood or tissue extracts and also containing neomycin and/or vancomycin. Strict anaerobiosis is essential for their recovery.

Bacteroides fragilis, a nonpleomorphic, saccharolytic organism with wide variations in biochemical characteristics, is a thin, gram-negative rod with rounded ends. This organism is probably the predominant member of the genus, but B. *funduliformis* is the species most frequently implicated in disease. It is pleomorphic and may appear as a small, thin, straight, or slightly curved rod; staining may be uniform, or bipolar granules may be observed. There are at least 30 known species of *Bacteroides*, but all may be considered to initiate disease in an approximately similar fashion.

Although generally considered nonpathogenic, bacteroides can cause disease in healthy young adults as well as in patients with underlying diseases or who have undergone recent trauma, surgery, or clinical manipulation. Bacteroides most frequently cause septicemia or abscess formation and have been found in gangrenous diseases of many types, often in association with other anaerobes, especially anaerobic streptococci. Thrombophlebitis at the site of the initial infection or of metastases is a hallmark of bacteroides infection. Septicemia most commonly arises from a primary

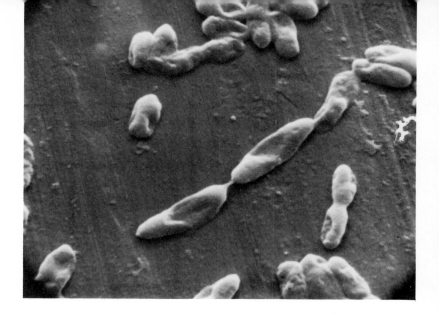

Fig. 14–1.
Bacteroides fragilis: Scanning electron micrograph. (×10,000)

lesion in the nasopharynx, lungs, intestine, appendix, genitourinary organs, or wounds.

Bacteroides infection of the lungs and pleural space is manifested by foul-smelling, occasionally blood-streaked, purulent sputum or pus. In patients with empyema, chest films may show gas above the pleural exudate as a result of the voluminous gas production characteristic of this organism. Here, too, mixed infections are common.

Postoperative wound infections are a significant problem; these are generally characterized by "bruising" about the incision, necrosis, venous thrombosis, foul-smelling purulent discharge, sinus formation, and metastatic abscesses. Well encapsulated hepatic abscesses have occurred in association with cholangitis; these must be differentiated from abscesses due to amebiasis, actinomycosis, or staphylococcal and streptococcal infections.

The diagnosis of bacteroides infection is frequently difficult. Strict anaerobiosis is necessary for culture, and sufficient growth for identification may not occur for several weeks. Immediate diagnosis therefore depends on clinical evidence and suspicion. Clues to diagnosis are: 1) foul-smelling pus containing gram-negative anaerobic rods, 2) classic symptoms of septicemia with no growth in blood cultures within the first 48–72 hours, 3) the presence of local thrombophlebitis, 4) the presence of gas-containing abscesses, and 5) unexplained postoperative fever following colonic surgery.

Therapy, which must be initiated before positive cultures are available, consists of open treatment of surgical wounds, prompt surgical drainage of abscesses, supportive therapy, and antibiotics.

SUGGESTED READING

1. BODNER SJ, KOENIG MG, GOODMAN JS: Bacteremic bacteroides infections. Ann Intern Med 73:537–544, 1970
2. FELNER JM, DOWELL VR: "Bacteroides" bacteremia. Am J Med 50:787–796, 1971

15

Other Gram-Negative Organisms

There are several other genera of gram-negative bacteria that are of medical importance to man.

FUSOBACTERIA All fusiform-shaped bacteria are not fusobacteria. This genus contains two major species: *Fusobacterium fusiforme and F. girans. F. fusiforme* is the more common species. It is a gram-negative, nonmotile, nonencapsulated, anaerobic or microaerophilic rod; it may be clear, granular, or filamentous with regularly disposed granules. Smooth colonies may show only uniform bacilli with tapering pointed ends appearing singly, in pairs, or in bundles resembling sheaves; rough colonies show a predominance of filaments. The organism produces indole and hydrogen sulfide, and therefore, a foul odor. Culture requires enriched media containing serum or ascitic fluid and generally a 2- to 5-day period for initial growth. After their initial isolation, many strains grow within 24 hours in thioglycollate broth without enrichment. The organism occurs naturally in the mouth, throat, intestine, and on the external genitalia.

F. girans is a gram-negative, strictly anaerobic, slender, pleomorphic bacillus with pointed ends (Fig. 15-1); it occasionally occurs as filaments and is characterized by a peculiar, elusive gyratory motility. It occurs naturally in the mouth and intestine. This organism requires enriched media for growth and produces neither indole nor hydrogen sulfide.

Fig. 15–1.
Fusobacterium girans. Scanning electron micrograph demonstrating uniform shape with tapered, pointed ends. (×10,000)

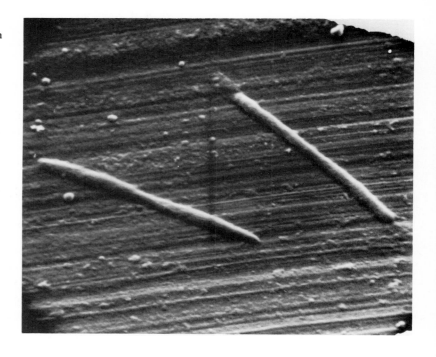

Perhaps the most common infection caused by fusiform bacilli is Vincent's angina or "trench mouth," generally a mixed infection of fusiform bacilli and oral spirochetes; the infection may progress by direct extension to involve the tonsils, sinus cavities, frontal bone, orbital cavities, and eye. Meningitis or brain abscesses represent direct extension rather than hematogenous spread. Fetid otitis or sinusitis should suggest fusobacterial infection. Disease originating in the gastrointestinal tract may lead to pyelophlebitis and peritonitis with metastases to the liver. Fusobacterial septicemia arising from the lungs originates from lower respiratory tract infection characterized by fetid sputum, hemoptysis, and often pulmonary gangrene or empyema. Fusobacterial septicemia has been reported after a human bite. Although infection with these organisms is uncommon, fusobacteria are typical of the unusual organisms encountered when host defenses are defective.

SPIRILLUM   The genus *Spirillum* consists of nine species of motile, spiral, gram-negative organisms, all but two of which are aerobic and grow well on artificial media. *Spirillum minus*, which cannot be artificially cultured, causes rat-bite fever (sodoku); the remaining species are generally considered nonpathogenic for man. These latter species have been recovered from stagnant water, putrified material, domestic animals, and fowl; in man they may be found in the nasopharynx, saliva, gingival crevices, on tooth surfaces, on external genitalia, and occasionally in feces.

Septicemia due to nonpathogenic spirilla has been reported in patients with altered host defenses. These infections often are associated with positive serologic tests for syphilis.

MIMEAE The tribe Mimeae includes two genera of clinical importance, *Mima* and *Herellea*, although the taxonomic relationships of this group of organisms remain unsettled. It is clinically convenient to classify all members as either *Mima polymorpha* or *Herellea vaginicola* according to their ability to ferment 10% lactose.

These organisms are pleomorphic (Fig. 15-2), gram-variable, non-pigmented, aerobic, nonsporulating, usually encapsulated, variably motile coccobacilli. Diplococcal forms predominate on solid media; rods and filaments are more conspicuous in liquid media. *M. polymorpha* ferments none of the common carbohydrates; *H. vaginicola* produces acid from glucose, galactose, xylose, arabinose, and 10% lactose, but not from 1% lactose, which is the standard concentration in routine laboratory use. This latter fermentation characteristic is extremely helpful in identification, and all unusual gram-negative organisms should be tested for their ability to ferment 10% lactose. These organisms are oxidase-negative except for a single species, *M. polymorpha* var. *oxidans*, which is oxidase-positive; the latter may cause confusion in distinguishing this group from the oxidase-positive neisseriae.

Mimeae classically are gram-negative but with a marked tendency toward gram-positivity. In smears of exudates the striking simultaneous presence of gram-positive and gram-negative diplococci, cocci in chains

Fig. 15–2.
Mima polymorpha. Scanning electron micrograph demonstrating pleomorphic coccobacillary form of the microorganisms. (×10,000)

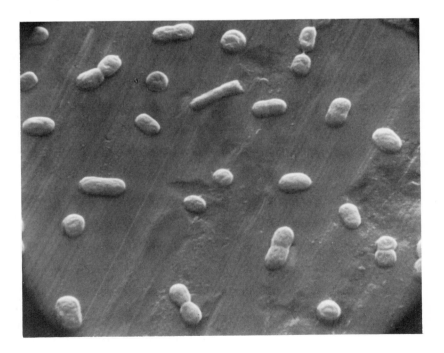

and clumps, pleomorphic rods, and coccobaccili should in itself suggest the presence of mimeae.

Members of this group may be found normally in the upper respiratory tract, sputum, feces, urine, vagina, urethra, external genitalia, and conjunctivae; about 25% of healthy persons carry *H. vaginicola* and 10% *M. polymorpha* somewhere on their skin surfaces.

Mimeae are not highly virulent or invasive under normal conditions and, except for meningitis and urethritis, cause apparent clinical infection most frequently in patients already seriously ill or debilitated by other diseases. Clinically, *M. polymorpha* and *H. vaginicola* cause similar diseases.

An increasing number of reports of *Mima* meningitis have appeared, and chronic meningitis has been recognized. Because this meningitis may occur with a diffuse petechial rash and overwhelming septicemia, it may be mistaken for meningococcal disease. Confusion is enhanced by the fact that mimeae may resemble gram-negative diplococci in smears. This presents a serious dilemma, since the treatment indicated for meningococcal meningitis is usually not the preferred therapy for mimeae infection. *Herellea* septicemia occurring in patients with underlying disease, recent surgery, or indwelling venous catheters has become an increasing problem.

Positive sputum cultures for mimeae and herelleae are frequent. Such findings need not reflect disease of the respiratory tract, although these organisms do cause bronchitis, pneumonia, lung abscess, and pleural effusion. They have also been implicated as respiratory pathogens in patients with cystic fibrosis.

As normal inhabitants of the urethra and vagina, these organisms complicate the diagnosis of gonorrhea by smear; some cases of "penicillin-resistant" gonorrhea may be due to mimeae and/or herelleae.

Although it is evident that members of the tribe Mimeae may cause disease of virtually every organ system, culture is necessary for identification. This group of organisms is becoming increasingly significant clinically; the frequency of isolation is often proportional to the awareness of the microbiologist of their occurrence and significance. Since their antibiotic sensitivity is variable, *in vitro* testing is mandatory. They are generally resistant to the usual doses of penicillin G and sulfonamides, a factor which makes differentiation from neisseriae of the utmost importance.

BRUCELLA   Brucellae are small, aerobic, gram-negative, nonmotile coccobacilli which are obligate intracellular parasites of man and animals. Typically *Brucella melitensis* infects goats, *B. abortus* cattle, and *B. suis* swine. In man brucellosis (undulant fever) presents as an acute febrile illness with bacteremia followed by a chronic indolent infection involving many tissues. The usual routes of infection whereby man contracts the disease from animals are the intestinal tract via the ingestion of infected milk, the mucous membranes via infected droplets, and the skin via direct contact with the tissues of infected animals. (Veterinarians are particularly susceptible to this mechanism of infection.) From the portal of entry, organisms spread to the lymphatics and regional lymph nodes and ultimately to the blood, with subsequent infection of the liver, spleen, bone marrow, and other parts of the reticuloendothelial system; granulomas and micro-abscesses are formed where the organisms maintain their intracellular location. Typical acute human brucellosis is characterized by fever, weakness, malaise, myalgia, arthralgia, lymphadenopathy, and hepatosplenomegaly that may last weeks or months. Chronic brucellosis follows with protean manifestations of obscure disease; diagnosis is difficult because organisms cannot be isolated during the chronic stage of brucellosis, but agglutinin titers may be high.

PASTEURELLA   Pasteurellae are short, aerobic or microaerophilic, gram-negative rods. *Pasteurella tularens* is the etiologic agent of tularemia, and *P. pestis* of plague.

Tularemia   *P. tularens* is a parasite of rodents; the reservoir of infection is maintained via transmission by the *Chrysops* fly and by ticks, especially *Dermacentor*. Man is infected mainly by skinning, handling, or eating infected rabbits and hares. The portals of entry are the skin or mucous membranes, gastrointestinal tract, respiratory route, or the opening made by the bites of arthropods. The site of penetration of the skin or mucous membranes is characterized by an ulcerating papule with enlargement and suppuration of the regional lymph nodes. Bacteremia results, with subsequent infection of many tissues and organs and the institution of granulomatous necrotic lesions. Three clinical types of tularemia are seen: 1) oculoglandular secondary to infection through the conjunctivae, 2) ulceroglandular following infection through the skin, and 3) pneumonic following pulmonary infection. In some cases the disease is limited to the lesion at the portal of entry; in others tularemia may present as fever of obscure etiology with no localizing symptoms or signs. It should be mentioned that *P. tularens*, the etiologic agent of tularemia, recently was reclassified and renamed *Francisella tularensis*.

Plague   *P. pestis* is a parasite of rodents, squirrels, and rats. Transmission among these hosts occurs via the bites of fleas, who were themselves infected by sucking the blood of infected animals. It is, however, rarely transmitted from man to man by fleas, but rather via droplet from human carriers or from cases of human infection with pneumonia. Pneumonic plague is a highly virulent disease that is almost always fatal if not immediately recognized and treated. If *P. pestis* infects man via the mucous membranes or skin, rapid enlargement of regional lymph nodes occurs to form a bubo (usually in the groin or axilla), which then undergoes necrosis and results in bubonic plague; infection may remain limited to the lymph nodes or spread to the blood with rapid dissemination of the organism.

SUGGESTED READING

1. DALY KA, POSTIC B, KASS EH: Infections due to organisms of the genus Herellae. Arch Intern Med 110:86–97, 1962

2. ELBERG SS: The brucellae, Bacterial and Mycotic Infections of Man. Fourth edition. Edited by RJ Dubos and JG Hirsch. Philadelphia, Lippincott, 1965, p 698

3. GREEN GS, JOHNSON RH, SHIVELY JA: Mimeae: opportunistic pathogens. JAMA 194: 163–166, 1965

4. HERMANN G, MELNICK T: Mima polymorpha meningitis in the young. Am J Dis Child 110:315–318, 1965

5. KLAINER AS, BEISEL WR: Opportunistic infections: a review. Am J Med Sci 258:431–456, 1969

6. MEYER KF: Pasteurella and francisella, Bacterial and Mycotic Infections of Man. Fourth edition. Edited by RJ Dubos and JG Hirsch. Philadelphia, Lippincott, 1965, p 659

16

Antimicrobial Agents

Antimicrobial agents* for therapy of infections are in common and widespread use. Their spectra of action, toxicities, pharmacologic properties, and various other facts are well documented; this information, beyond the scope of this book, can be found in a variety of texts. This chapter is meant merely to summarize and illustrate the mechanism of action of the common antimicrobial agents.

Antimicrobial agents differ markedly in mechanisms of action, just as they do in various other properties. The common antimicrobial drugs listed in Table 16–1 fall into five distinct categories, illustrating that these drugs act on many sites of the microbial cell. Regardless of the actual mechanism involved, however, all are active because each interferes with, or affects in a deleterious way, some vital biochemical cellular process. Elucidation of these mechanisms (Fig. 16-1) at a molecular or fundamental level required sophisticated biochemical techniques. The effect an antimicrobial agent has on the microbial cell is hidden deeply within the cell. Except for one mode of action there are no visible external changes. Microorganisms susceptible to the action of antimicrobial agents which

---

* In common usage, "antimicrobial agent" and "antibiotic" are synonymous terms, but such usage lacks precision. The term antibiotic should be reserved for substances of microbial origin which act on other microorganisms by suppressing their growth. In contrast, antimicrobial agent is a broader term; it includes antibiotics and compounds synthesized in the laboratory. Regardless of the origin, these materials act either by suppressing growth or by killling microorganisms.

DIAGRAMMATIC REPRESENTATIONS OF MECHANISMS OF ACTION OF SELECTED ANTIMICROBIAL AGENTS

I Griseofulvin blocks DNA synthesis. The molecular structure of griseofulvin is analogous to the purine nucleosides.

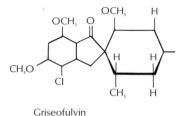

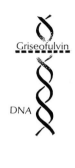

Griseofulvin

Guanoside

II Antimicrobial agents which interfere with protein synthesis

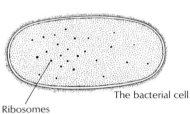

Ribosomes
sites of protein synthesis

The bacterial cell

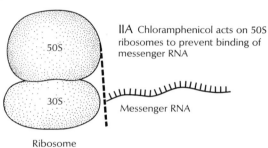

IIA Chloramphenicol acts on 50S ribosomes to prevent binding of messenger RNA

Messenger RNA

Ribosome

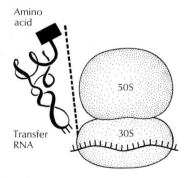

IIB Tetracycline binds to 30S ribosome to prevent access of amino-acyl transfer RNA.

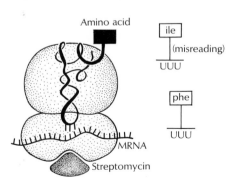

IIC Streptomycin acts on the ribosome to cause misreading of genetic code. (UUU which codes for phenylalanine (phe) may code for isoleucine (ile) instead)

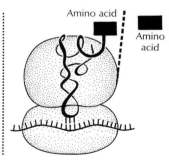

IID Erythromycin binds to 50S ribosome to suppress polypeptide polymerization (amino acid linkages)

Fig. 16–1.
Mechanism of action of selected antimicrobial agents.

III Sulfonamides interfere with intermediate metabolism

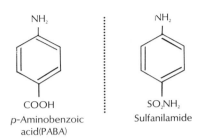

p-Aminobenzoic
acid(PABA)

Sulfanilamide

Sulfonamides are structural analogs for p-aminobenzoic acid (PABA), a component of folic acid, itself a component of purine synthesis. The sulfonamides are competitive antagonists of PABA, or form false folic acid.

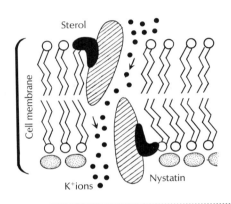

IV Nystatin binds to the sterol moiety in the cell membrane of sensitive fungi. Changes in permeability allows leakage of potassium ions and other cellular components

V Penicillin interferes with the final stage of cell wall synthesis

Penicillin, acting as a structual analog of D-alanyl-D-alanine (lower right), blocks cross linking of peptide side chains in the mucopeptide layer of the bacterial wall.

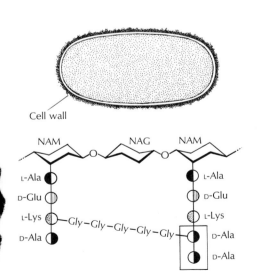

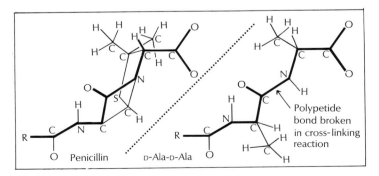

Table 16-1. Mechanisms of Antimicrobial Action

Interfere with cell wall synthesis
    Penicillins
    Cephalosporins
    Cycloserine
    Vancomycin
    Ristocetin
    Bacitracin
Affect cell membrane (detergent effect)
    Polymyxins
    Colistin
    Novobiocin
    Polyene antifungal agents (nystatin, amphotericin)
Interfere with intracellular protein synthesis
    Chloramphenicol
    Tetracyclines
    Kanamycin
    Neomycin
    Gentamicin
    Streptomycins
    Macrolide antibiotics (erythromycin, troleandomycin)
Affect nucleic acid metabolism
    Griseofulvin
Affect intermediary metabolism
    Sulfonamides
    Isoniazid
    Aminosalicylic acid
    Ethambutol

Fig. 16–2.
Staphylococcus aureus, untreated cells. (Klainer AS, Betsch CJ: J Infect Dis 121:339–343, Copyright [1970] The University of Chicago) (×10,000)

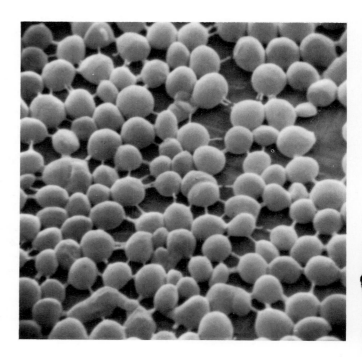

Fig. 16–3.

Staphylococcus aureus treated with cephalothin, 0.1 MIC (minimum inhibitory concentration) for 90 minutes. "Blebs" on the surfaces of some cells are consistent with drug-induced defects in the cell wall; irregular spherical structures lying free or appearing to extrude from cells are also seen. (Klainer AS, Perkins RL: Hosp Pract 4:88–97, 1971) (×10,000)

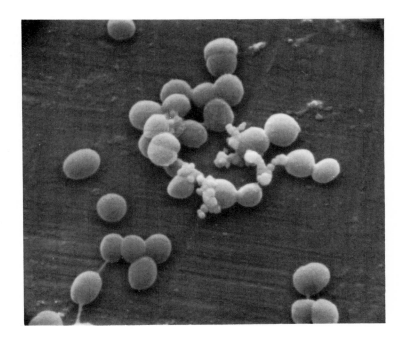

interfere with biochemical (enzymatic) reactions responsible for cell wall synthesis develop alterations in their cell surfaces. These are readily visible and have become highly significant for an understanding of cell wall-active substances.

Although a great deal of information on the mode of action of cell wall-active agents was obtained with optical microscopes, progress was accelerated when the scanning electron microscope became available. This instrument is peculiarly suitable for studying surface details of any substance. It has been used with singular results in elucidating the surface morphology of microorganisms and the effect of antimicrobial agents thereon. The effects of three cell wall-active antimicrobial drugs—cephalothin, penicillin G, and carbenicillin—on the morphology of *Staphylococcus aureus, Escherichia coli,* and *Pseudomonas aeruginosa,* respectively, are illustrated in Figures 16-2 through 16-22.

Staphylococcus aureus. Normal untreated cells of *S. aureus* are spherical with smooth surfaces and are arranged in typical grape-like clusters (Fig. 16-2). Upon exposure of normal penicillin-sensitive cells to increased concentrations of cephalothin or penicillin G, surface defects begin to appear (Fig. 16-3); small bleb-like imperfections can be seen on a few cells, and irregularly spherical masses resembling granules lie free or seem to extrude from cells. As more defects occur the cell wall becomes less able to maintain the size and shape of some cells, and this combination of multiple surface defects and increase in size results in a "raspberry" or "cobblestone" appearance (Fig. 16-4). Then larger cells appear, as do cells considerably

Fig. 16–4.
Staphylococcus aureus treated with cephalothin, 1.0 MIC for 90 minutes. There are cells with multiple surface defects resulting in a "raspberry" or "cobblestone" appearance. (Klainer AS, Perkins RL: J Infect Dis 122:323–328, Copyright [1970] The University of Chicago) (×10,000)

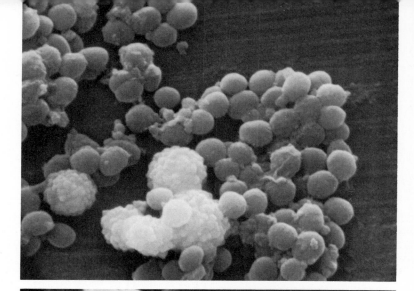

Fig. 16–5 and 16–6.
Staphylococcus aureus treated with cephalothin, 1.0 MIC for 90 minutes (×10,000). Cells with defects previously described are seen, as are somewhat larger cells with a mosaic surface and large smooth cells consistent with spheroplasts. (Klainer AS, Perkins RL: J Infect Dis 122:323–328, Copyright [1970] The University of Chicago) (×20,000)

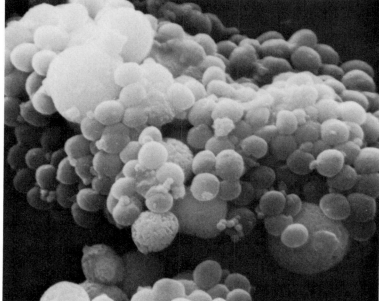

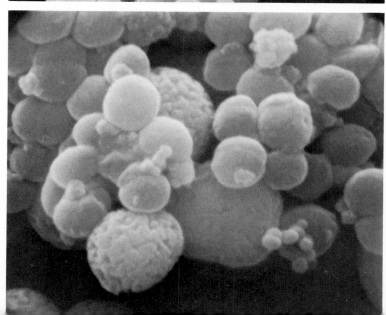

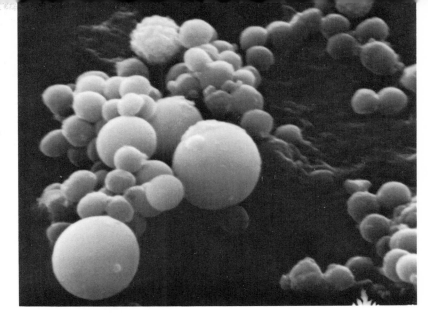

Fig. 16–7 and 16–8.
Staphylococcus aureus treated with
cephalothin, 1.0 MIC for 90
minutes. Large smooth cells
consistent with spheroplasts are
present. (Klainer AS, Perkins RL:
JAMA 215:1655–1657, 1971)
(×10,000)

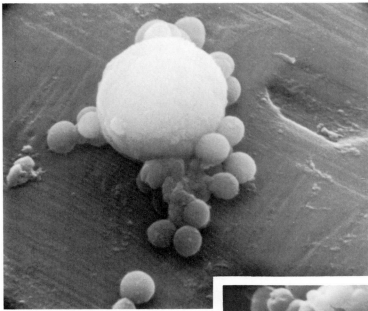

Fig. 16–9.
Staphylococcus aureus. These are
large irregular forms consistent with
cell wall-defective staphylococci.
Note discrete defects on the surface
of this cell. (Klainer AS, Perkins RL:
JAMA 215:1655–1657, 1971)
(×10,000)

Fig. 16–10.
Streptococcus pyogenes. Right: Untreated control. Left: After treatment with cephalothin there is swelling of the cells with defects at midcell resembling an apple core. (Klainer AS, Perkins RL: Hosp Pract 4:88–97, 1971) (×10,000)

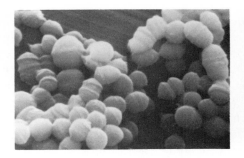 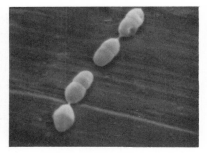

Fig. 16–11.
Escherichia coli, untreated cells. (×10,000)

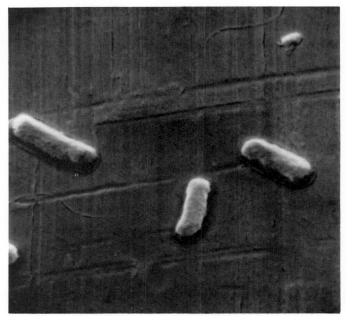

Fig. 16–12.
Escherichia coli treated with 0.1 MIC penicillin G for three hours. Note elongation presumably due to interference with cell division but not cell growth. (Klainer AS, Perkins RL: JAMA 215:1655–1657, 1971) (×2,000)

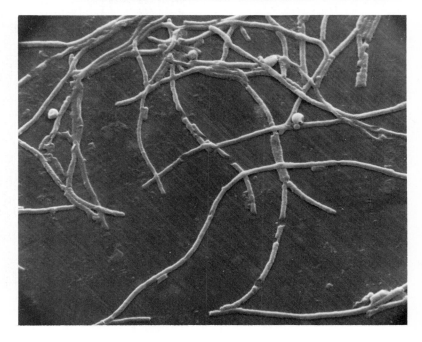

more symmetrical in form and characterized by a mosaic-like surface pattern (Figs. 16-5 and 16-6). Finally greatly enlarged cells with essentially smooth surfaces (Figs. 16-7 and 16-8) are seen; these may become distorted and appear as large, irregularly shaped forms with discrete surface defects (Fig. 16-9), resembling typical cell wall-defective *S. aureus* or "L-forms."

Figure 16-10 illustrates the effect of cephalothin on group A β-hemolytic streptococci and demonstrates a somewhat different morphologic change. In this case defects occur mainly at midcell at the site of new cell wall synthesis causing the treated cells to enlarge and develop an apple core appearance.

Exposure of penicillin-resistant *S. aureus* to penicillin G results in no demonstrable changes. The effect of cephalothin, however, is similar (as described) in both penicillin-sensitive and penicillin-resistant organisms, reflecting the resistance of the cephalosporins to the action of penicillinase, an enzyme which inactivates penicillin and is characteristic of many penicillin-resistant bacteria.

Escherichia coli. Normal untreated cells of *E. coli* resemble cylinders or rods of various lengths with somewhat irregular surfaces (Fig. 16-11); the ends are typically rounded but may be flattened, a result of preparation of the specimen for scanning electron microscopic examination. When normal cells are exposed to increasing concentrations of either cephalothin or penicillin G, the cells first elongate to many times their usual length (Fig. 16-12); this occurs because low concentrations of these drugs inhibit

Fig. 16–13.
Escherichia coli treated with penicillin, 0.1 MIC for 90 minutes, during its logarithmic phase of growth resulting in a tubular outpouching from the cell wall. (Klainer AS, Perkins RL: J Infect Dis 122:323–328, Copyright [1970] The University of Chicago) (×10,000)

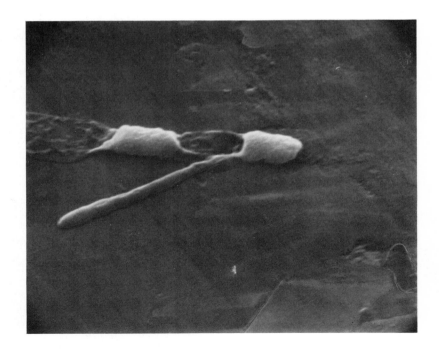

Fig. 16–14.
Escherichia coli treated with 1.0 MIC penicillin G for three hours. Note single defect at midcell and flattened cell membranes in background. (Klainer AS, Perkins RL: JAMA 215:1655–1657, 1971) (×10,000)

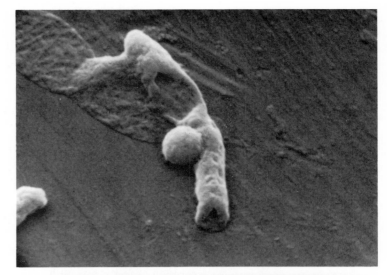

Fig. 16–15.
Escherichia coli treated with penicillin, 1 MIC for 90 minutes, during its logarithmic phase of growth. (Klainer AS, Perkins RL: J Infect Dis 122:323–328, Copyright [1970] The University of Chicago) (×20,000)

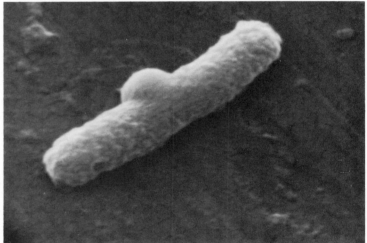

Fig. 16–16.
Escherichia coli treated with 1.0 MIC penicillin G for three hours. Note enlarging defect at midcell at site of transverse septum formation. (Klainer AS, Perkins RL: JAMA 215:1655–1657, 1971) (×10,000)

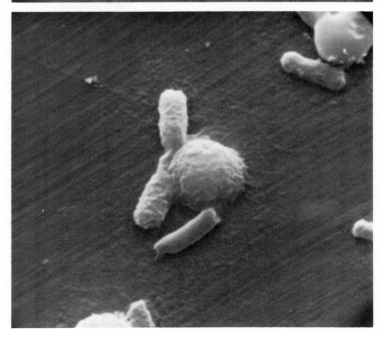

Fig. 16–17.
Escherichia coli treated with 10 MIC
penicillin G for three hours. Note large
collapsed defect at midcell. (Klainer AS,
Perkins RL: JAMA 215:1655–1657,
1971) (×20,000)

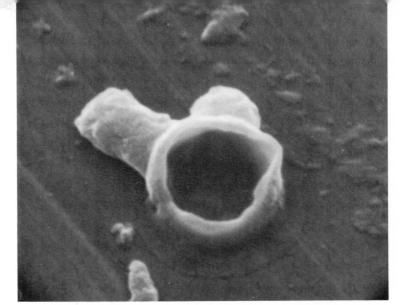

Fig. 16–18.
Escherichia coli treated with 10 MIC
penicillin G for three hours. Note
spectrum of drug effect from intact cells
in midfield to intact and collapsed
spheroplasts in periphery. (Klainer AS,
Perkins RL: JAMA 215:1655–1657,
1971) (×5,000)

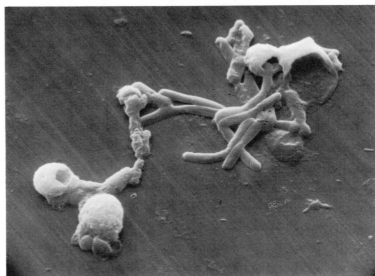

Fig. 16–19.
Escherichia coli, showing a spectrum of
drug effects including grossly unaffected
cells, spherical forms consistent with
spheroplasts, and collapsed forms
consistent with cell membranes. (Klainer
AS, Perkins RL: J Infect Dis 122:323–
328, Copyright [1970] The University of
Chicago) (×5,000)

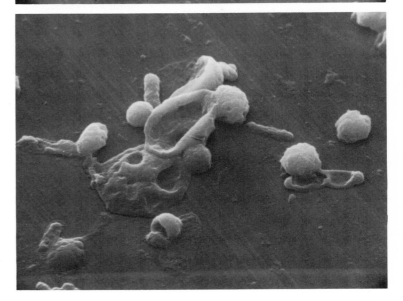

cell division but not cell growth, and the cell continues to grow, i.e., elongate, but not divide. An additional defect which occurs in some cells at low drug concentrations is the spherical pouch-like protrusion seen in Figures 16-13 through 16-15; the defect is at midcell, the site of transverse septum formation and the weakest part of the cell wall. The defect enlarges in cells exposed to larger concentrations of drugs (Fig. 16-16) and may collapse (Fig. 16-17). The spectrum of antibiotic effect is seen in Figure 16-18 and 16-19, which demonstrate normal-appearing and elongated cells, some surface defects, various sizes of saccular pouch-like protrusions located at midcell, and large, approximately spherical forms called spheroplasts which appear intact or in a state of collapse.

Pseudomonas aeruginosa. Figures 16-20 through 16-22 demonstrate the effects of carbenicillin. In very sensitive organisms defects occur at many sites on the surface of the cell (Fig. 16-21), but only at the sensitive midcell site in a more resistant strain (Fig. 16-22).

The morphologic changes which occur in *S. aureus*, *E. coli*, and *Ps. aeruginosa* as a result of exposure to cephalothin, penicillin G, or carbenicillin, respectively, are a visual representation of the mechanism of action of cell wall-active antimicrobial agents. The stepwise progression from normal to abnormal morphology differs in some details for different organisms. Nevertheless, the structure which finally emerges in each case is comparable. This structure is the spheroplast, a cell which no longer has an intact cell wall. It is incapable of maintaining its classic size and shape and thus is no longer morphologically recognizable as *S. aureus*, *E. coli*, or *Ps. aeruginosa*. Furthermore, in an environment which is entirely satisfactory for cells with normal morphology, the spheroplast swells and finally bursts.

The morphologic alterations of these organisms have been observed only *in vitro*. A similar series of changes is postulated to occur *in vivo* during therapy with these antibiotics. Accordingly, it may be assumed that spheroplasts—possibly cells with lesser defects—do not find the host's milieu a favorable environment and by swelling and bursting meet destruction.

The mechanisms of action of antimicrobial agents which act other than on cell wall synthesis do not lend themselves well to photographic illustration. These have been graphically summarized in Figure 16-1, and more complete descriptions are presented in other texts and articles. It should be emphasized, however, that the proper use of antimicrobial therapy in the treatment of infectious diseases requires not only knowledge of the basic mechanism of actions of these drugs and their pharmacology but, more important, extensive experience. This chapter is meant only as a brief descriptive introduction.

SUGGESTED READING

1. WEINSTEIN L: Chemotherapy of microbial diseases, The Pharmacologic Basis of Therapeutics. Fourth edition. Edited by LS Goodman and A Gilman. New York, MacMillan, 1970, pp 1154–1343

Fig. 16–20.
Pseudomonas aeruginosa, untreated cells.
(×10,000)

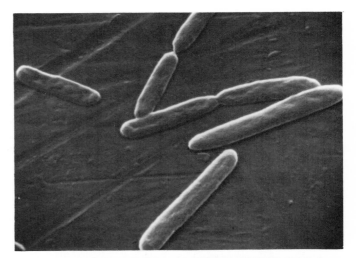

Fig. 16–21.
Pseudomonas aeruginosa: a sensitive strain treated
with carbenicillin, 1.0 MIC for 90 minutes.
Note the multiple discrete saccular defects along
the surface of the cell. (Klainer AS, Perkins RL:
J Infect Dis 122:323–328, Copyright [1970] The
University of Chicago) (×20,000)

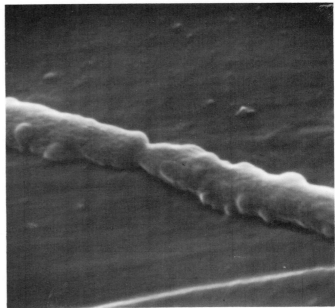

Fig. 16–22.
Pseudomonas aeruginosa: a more
resistant strain than that in Figure
16–21, treated with 10 MIC
carbenicillin for 2 hours, demonstrating
a single large defect at midcell at the
site of transverse septum formation.
(×20,000)

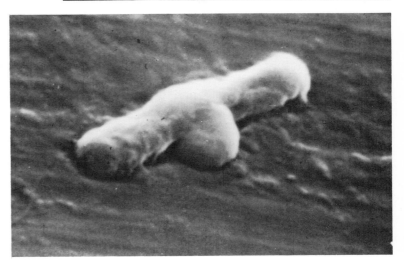

Index

Oxidase test, for gonococci, 85
Oxidative phosphorylation, volutin granules and, 11
Oxygen, bacterial requirements for, 31

P-ring
  of basal body, 11, *13*
Palisade arrangement, in bacteria, 20, 91, 105
Paracolon bacilli, classification of, 119–120
Parasites
  extracellular, 35
  intracellular, 35
  nutritional requirements of, 30
Paratyphoids A, B, and C, classification of, 126
Passive immunity, definition of, 43
Passive transport, by cell membranes, 9, 10
Pasteurella pestis, plague from, 139
Pasteurella tularens, tularemia from, 139
Pasteurellae
  characteristics and pathogenicity of, 139
  plague from, 139
  tularemia from, 139
Penicillin(s)
  in diphtheria therapy, 94
  effects on cell wall, 4, 145, 148, 149–152
  in gas gangrene therapy, 101
  in gonorrhea therapy, 84, 88, 89
  mechanism of action of, 143, 144
    on E. coli, *148, 149, 150–151,* 152
    on S. aureus, 145, 148
  in pneumococcal pneumonia therapy, 71
  in tetanus therapy, 100
Penicillin G
  effects on *E. coli, 148, 149, 150–151,* 152
  mimae resistance to, 138
  S. aureus resistance to, 149
Perihepatitis, gonococcal, 87
Perinephric abscess, staphylococcal, 65
Peritonitis, pneumococcal, 70
Peritrichous flagella, *13*
  definition of, 13
Pertussis vaccine, in DPT toxoids, 95, 116
pH, bacterial requirements for, 31

Phagocytes
  microscopy of, *40–42*
  types of, 38
Phagocytosis
  bacterial defense against, 37
  definition of, 38
  diagram of, 39
  function of, 38, 43
  impaired, in diabetes, 52
  stages in, 38
Pharyngitis
  membranous
    causes of, 93
    in diphtheria, 93, 94
  streptococcal, 77, 79, 93
Phase microscopy, of bacteria, 26, 28
Phenylbutazone, effects on phagocytosis, 54
Phosphate, bacterial need for, 32
Phosphatidyl choline, in cell membrane, 8
Phospholipid, in endotoxins, 36
Picket-fence arrangement, in bacteria, 20, 91
Pili, structure and function of, 14
Pituitary gland, phagocytic cells in, 38
Placenta, infection transfer by, 46
Plague, symptoms and etiology of, 139
Pneumococci, 67–72
  antigenic structure of, 70
  axes of, 20, 67, 69
  C-substance of, 70
  capsules of, 70
  cultural characteristics of, 70
  as diplococci, 20
  diseases from, 70–72
  immunity to, 72
  M-protein of, 70
  morphology of, 17, 18, 67
  R-antigen of, 70
  spatial arrangement of, 20
  streptococci compared to, 76
  tissue invasion by, 35
  vaccines for, 72
Pneumococcus, capsule of, 1, 4
Pneumocystis, as opportunistic invader, 55
Pneumonia
  enteric, 119
  from *Klebsiella*, 120
  pneumococcal, 67, 68, 70, 71, 72, 116
  staphylococcal, 60, 64–65, 116
Pneumonic plague, symptoms and etiology of, 139
Polyhydroxybutyric acid, in storage granules, 11

Polymetaphosphates, in storage granules, 11
Polymyxins, mechanism of action of, 144
Polymorphonuclear leukocytes
  in detection of opportunistic bacteria, 57
  as phagocytes, *39–42*
  in pneumococcal pneumonia, 72
Polypeptide
  of bacterial capsule, 1
  of bacterial cell wall, 8
Polyribosomes, in cytoplasm, 11
Polysaccharide
  of bacterial capsules, 1, 120
  in endotoxins, 36
Potassium
  bacterial need for, 32
  deficiency, infection following, 52
Precipitins, antibody activity of, 42
Pregnancy
  coliform urinary infection in, 123
  listeriosis in, 107
  pneumococcal pneumonia in, 71
Prostheses, as factors in opportunistic infections, 50, 51, 54
Protein
  deficiency, opportunistic infection in, 53
  intracellular synthesis of, antimicrobial interference with, 142, 144
Proteinase, streptococcal, 78
Proteus
  classification of, 119, 120
  endotoxin shock from, 36
  flagella of, 14
  as opportunistic invader, 55
  urinary infections from, 124
Proteus mirabilis
  classification of, 124
  phagocytosis of, *41*
  in urinary infection, 123, 124
Proteus morgani, classification of, 124
Proteus rettgeri, classification of, 124
Proteus vulgaris
  cell wall of, environment effects on, 5
  classification of, 124
  flagella of, *12*
  morphology of, *125*
Pseudomonas
  classification of, 119, 120, 124
  as opportunistic invader, 55
  pathogenicity of, 124
  urinary infection from, 123
Pseudomonas aeruginosa
  antimicrobial agent effects on, 145, 152, *153*

Text design and layout by Maria S. Karkucinski

Composition in Electra, linotype,
American Book–Stratford Press, Inc.
Printed by Murray Printing Co.

Harper & Row, Publishers

73 74 75 76 77 78 10 9 8 7 6 5 4 3 2 1

DATE DUE